FUNDAMENTALS
OF CLINICAL
PSYCHOPHARMACOLOGY

Fourth Edition

Edited by

Ian M Anderson MA MD MRCP(UK) FRCPsych
Professor of Psychiatry
Neuroscience and Psychiatry Unit
The University of Manchester
Manchester, UK

R Hamish McAllister-Williams MD PhD FRCPsych
Reader in Clinical Psychopharmacology
Institute of Neuroscience
Newcastle University
Newcastle upon Tyne, UK

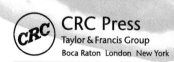

CRC Press
Taylor & Francis Group
Boca Raton London New York

CRC Press is an imprint of the
Taylor & Francis Group, an **informa** business

CRC Press
Taylor & Francis Group
6000 Broken Sound Parkway NW, Suite 300
Boca Raton, FL 33487-2742

Printed on acid-free paper
Version Date: 20150713

International Standard Book Number-13: 978-1-4987-1894-3 (Paperback)

Visit the Taylor & Francis Web site at
http://www.taylorandfrancis.com

and the CRC Press Web site at
http://www.crcpress.com

Printed and bound by CPI Group (UK) Ltd, Croydon, CR0 4YY

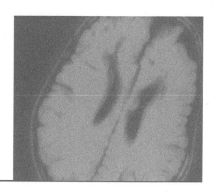

This book is dedicated to the memory of Ian Reid who died prematurely in 2014 after a short illness. He was co-editor of the first three editions of *Fundamentals* and a contributor to a number of chapters. Without him the earlier editions, and therefore this one, would not have been published. Ian was proud to have been one of the first to propose the neurotrophic and neuroplasticity hypothesis of antidepressant action and was well known for his fierce intelligence, wit and iconoclasm. You can read more about Ian in the BAP December 2014 newsletter (http://www.bap.org.uk/pdfs/BAPNewsletterDec2014.pdf). He is greatly missed on both a professional and a personal level.

Contents

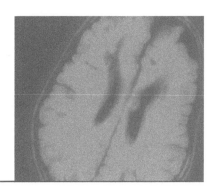

Foreword

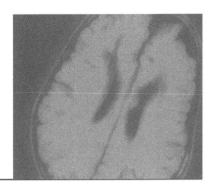

It is a pleasure to write the foreword to this welcome, and much antici-pated, new edition of *Fundamentals*. The book is a key component of the British Association for Psychopharmacology (BAP)'s commitment to ensuring that accurate, evidence-based and unbiased information about psychopharmacology is available to a wide audience through a variety of activities and media. True to the BAP ethos, the book spans the range of the discipline, from the mode of action and side effects of drugs, via key aspects of the biology of psychiatric disorders, to meta-analyses of clinical trials. Wherever possible, it is anchored to the practice guidelines produced by the UK National Institute for Health and Care Excellence (NICE) and the BAP itself. The editors and authors are to be commended for bring-ing together such a comprehensive and up-to-date book that will be of particular use to trainees and consultant psychiatrists, as well as to other mental health professionals and physicians, both in their day-to-day prac-tice and as an accessible and concise reference volume. I also echo the authors' dedication and gratitude to the late Ian Reid for his critical role in co-editing and contributing to the earlier editions.

There is no other area of medicine where a book such as this, summaris-ing the science behind, and the practice of, therapeutic prescribing could be seen as anything other than of value and importance. Yet there is a con-tinuing view held by a vociferous minority that the drugs used in psychiatry are at best ineffective, at worst dangerous, and that their use is usually, if not always, inappropriate. Moreover, those who carry out research in, or are supportive of, psychopharmacology, are often portrayed as being in the pocket of the pharmaceutical industry. Any rational reading of the current text, or perusal of the author list, shows that such views are unsustainable and unfair. Yet the criticisms do highlight the need for all of us who advo-cate that medication has an important place in the treatment of people with mental health disorders, to ensure that our actions and opinions are justified, and with transparency regarding any real or perceived conflicts of interest. Certainly, it is crucial that anyone prescribing psychotropic medication does so with a solid grounding in the underlying science and clinical evidence, and that they present the case for, and against, medication in a balanced fashion to patients[1]. But these principles apply equally to those studying or advocating psychological or other interventions; these are also susceptible to bias, error and conflicts – albeit often overlooked and less clearly delineated[2].

The real argument in favour of psychopharmacology is, however, that drugs work, and with effect sizes comparable to those in general medicine[3]. Nor should we be defensive about comparisons with psychological treatment[4]. For example, using like-for-like methodology, antidepressants have at least comparable clinical benefit to psychological treatments for depression, even after taking into account unpublished drug studies[5,6]. In the acute treatment of schizophrenia, drug treatments have moderate-to-large effects, whereas an addition of cognitive therapy adds only a small-to-moderate benefit, which is lower in the more methodologically rigorous studies[7,8]. In essence, whether one views the psychopharmacological glass as half full or half empty, an equally critical conclusion should be drawn with regard to psychotherapies.

None of these points are intended to downplay the place of psychological treatments in psychiatry – they work too and are often preferred by patients – but rather to highlight that all patients deserve clear and accurate advice about, and access to, effective psychopharmacological *and* psychological treatments. In this context, the new edition of *Fundamentals* provides a balanced and valuable summary of the evidence for the efficacy, indications and mechanisms of action of current psychotropic drugs. It will be of wide clinical value, as well as provide a clear synthesis of the psychopharmacological evidence, and a defence against misplaced or unfounded criticisms.

Paul J Harrison
Professor of Psychiatry
University of Oxford
Oxford, United Kingdom
President
British Association for Psychopharmacology
Cambridge, United Kingdom

 ## References

1. Harrison PJ, Baldwin DS, Barnes TRE et al. No psychiatry without psychopharmacology. *Br J Psychiatry* 2011; 199: 263–265.
2. Nutt DJ, Sharpe M. Uncritical positive regard? Issues in the efficacy and safety of psychotherapy. *J Psychopharmacol* 2008; 22: 3–6.

3. Leucht S, Hierl S, Kissling W. Putting the efficacy of psychiatric and general medicine medication into perspective: Review of meta-analyses. *Br J Psychiatry* 2012;
200: 97–106.
4. Huhn M, Tardy M, Spinelli LM et al. Efficacy of pharmacotherapy and psychotherapy for adult psychiatric disorders: A systematic overview of meta-analyses. *JAMA
Psychiatry* 2014; 71: 706–715.
5. Turner EH, Matthews AM, Linardatos E et al. Selective publication of antidepressant trials and its influence on apparent efficacy. *N Engl J Med.* 2008; 358: 252–260.
6. Cuijpers P, Turner EH, Mohr DC et al. Comparison of psychotherapies for adult
depression to pill placebo control groups: A meta-analysis. *Psychol Med.* 2014; 44:
685–695.
7. Leucht S, Cipriani A, Spineli L. Comparative efficacy and tolerability of 15 antipsychotic drugs in schizophrenia: A multiple-treatments meta-analysis. *Lancet.* 2013;
382: 951–962.
8. Jauhar S, McKenna PJ, Radua J. Cognitive-behavioural therapy for the symptoms of
schizophrenia: Systematic review and meta-analysis with examination of potential bias. *Br J Psychiatry.* 2014; 204: 20–29.

Preface

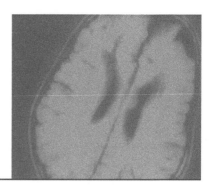

It is 13 years since the first edition of *Fundamentals of Clinical Psychopharmacology* was published in 2002. It was intended to be a frequently updated, affordable, concise and practical textbook that would meet the needs of trainees and practitioners seeking to keep abreast of the state of the art of psychopharmacology. After further editions in 2004 and 2006, why has there been a gap of nine years before this edition? The reasons have included a slowdown in drug development, translating into fewer clinically available new drugs, the financial and marketing environment (especially since 2008) and some revision fatigue on the part of editors and authors. We are therefore grateful to the publisher for wishing to undertake this new edition and for being willing to make it more affordable and therefore hopefully accessible to a wider audience, particularly trainees. We are also extremely grateful to the authors – both past and new contributors – for agreeing to provide their time and expertise. The *Fundamentals* developed from the British Association for Psychopharmacology (BAP)'s 'Psychopharmacology Course for Psychiatrists in Training', which has developed into the acclaimed current 'Masterclasses in Clinical Psychopharmacology' for all clinicians involved in prescribing. This book is part of the strong educational tradition of the BAP (see later for more details).

The remit of the book is to provide a core of up-to-date, clinically relevant information about drugs in the context of current knowledge about the biological basis of the disorders they treat. For this new edition, we have updated all the chapters and have included a new one on practical prescribing. It has allowed us to correct inevitable mistakes and we continue to put drug prescribing into the context of National Institute of Health and Care Excellence (NICE) guidance. As well as having obvious UK relevance, NICE remains the most influential, comprehensive and coherent authority producing evidence-based guidance across the world. However, guidance is increasingly being interpreted in a narrow way and can be employed as a restriction on choice rather than as an enabler of good practice. It is therefore vital to critically evaluate the evidence and at times adopt a healthy scepticism of guidelines, because of the complex procedures, and often political compromises, that lie behind them. As with previous editions, for ease of reading, we have not included in-text citations. Key references, including any clinical studies mentioned, are given at the end of each chapter together with additional further reading.

The current contributors to the book are leading psychopharmacologists, predominantly from the United Kingdom, but the content of the book has developed over subsequent editions and we must thank the many others who have been involved in the material over the years, and they are listed in the acknowledgements. We would particularly like to acknowledge the contribution of Prof Ian Reid, to whom this book is dedicated.

The BAP was founded in 1974, with the general intention of bringing together those from clinical and experimental disciplines, human- and animal-based research as well as members of the pharmaceutical industry involved in the study of psychopharmacology. It is one of the largest national associations of its kind in the world. The BAP arranges scientific meetings, fosters research and teaching, encourages the publication of research, produces clinical guidelines, publishes the *Journal of Psychopharmacology* and provides guidance and information to the public on matters relevant to psychopharmacology. BAP evidence-based guidelines are available for downloading for personal use from our website. The BAP has also produced an online continuing professional development (CPD) resource, which is frequently updated and expanded. This, together with the various face-to-face meetings organised by the BAP, is recommended to anyone wanting to gain further information beyond this book.

Membership of the BAP is open to anyone with a relevant degree related to neuroscience, including clinical medical, nursing, or pharmacy degrees. If you are interested in any aspect of psychopharmacology, we would strongly encourage you to consider joining. You can find out more on our website: http://www.bap.org.uk.

Ian M Anderson
R Hamish McAllister Williams
British Association for Psychopharmacology
Cambridge, United Kingdom

Acknowledgements

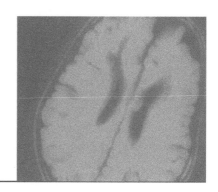

We thank the many people who have contributed to earlier editions or were involved in the development of the material:

Prof Clive Adams
Dr Harry Allen
Dr David Balfour
Prof Thomas Barnes
Dr Geoff Bennett
Prof Steve Cooper
Prof Philip Cowen
Prof Bill Deakin
Dr Colin Dourish
Prof Barry Everitt
Prof Nicol Ferrier
Dr Sophia Frangou
Prof Guy Goodwin
Prof Chris Hollis
Prof John Hughes

Prof Eileen Joyce
Prof Robert Kerwin
Prof David King
Prof Shôn Lewis
Dr Andrea Malizia
Dr Jan Melichar
Prof David Nutt
Prof Veronica O'Keane
Prof Carmine Pariante
Prof Lyn Pilowsky
Prof Ian Reid
Prof Craig Ritchie
Dr Clare Stanford
Dr Mike Travis
Dr Stuart Watson

Editors

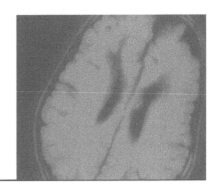

Prof Ian M Anderson, BA, MA, MBBS, MD, MRCP(UK), FRCPsych, is professor of psychiatry, Neuroscience and Psychiatry Unit, University of Manchester, and honorary consultant psychiatrist, Manchester Mental Health and Social Care Trust.

Prof Anderson founded the Specialist Service for Affective Disorders in Manchester and was director until 2011. His research interests include the aetiology and treatment of mood disorders, the mechanism of action of antidepressants and evidence-based psychiatry. He chaired the guideline development group for the 2009 update of the NICE depression clinical guideline and is an author on several consensus treatment guidelines from the British Association for Psychopharmacology (BAP). He is a past general secretary of the BAP.

Dr R Hamish McAllister-Williams, BSc, MBChB, PhD, MD, FRCPsych, is reader in clinical psychopharmacology, Institute of Neuroscience, Newcastle University, and honorary consultant psychiatrist, Regional Affective Disorders Service, Northumberland Tyne and Wear NHS Foundation Trust.

Dr McAllister-Williams is the lead consultant in the tertiary level Regional Affective Disorders Service based in Newcastle for patients with treatment-refractory mood disorders. His research focuses on the pathophysiology and treatment of both bipolar and unipolar affective disorders, and he is an author of the BAP consensus guidelines for treating depression. He is a past general secretary of the BAP and was appointed its director of education in 2012.

A note on nomenclature

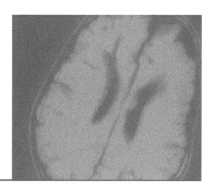

The current classification, or nomenclature, of psychotropic drugs can be unhelpful in understanding their pharmacology or clinical use. In clinical use, it has grown in a random way with inconsistencies in whether drugs are classified according to chemical structure, history, clinical effects or pharmacology. The World Health Organisation (WHO) system, the Anatomical Therapeutic Chemical Classification System (http://www.who.int/classifications/atcddd/en/), is a little better, with the division of drugs into different groups according to the organ or system on which they act and their chemical, pharmacological, and therapeutic properties. For example, antipsychotics are classified according to chemical structure but antidepressants according to pharmacology. Many drugs are listed under an 'other' category, and this can be a particular problem with newer compounds. In addition, drugs which act on a range of disorders sit uneasily in the current schemes (e.g. 'antidepressants' are also first-line drugs in treating anxiety disorders, and newer 'antipsychotics' are effective treatments for depression).

In response to this, a taskforce, supported by four major neuropsychopharmacology organisations, has proposed a multi-axial, pharmacologically driven nomenclature for psychiatric drugs (neuroscience-based nomenclature or 'NbNomenclature') that they have field-tested (http://www.ecnp.eu/projects-initiatives/nomenclature.aspx). The final published version has four axes. Axis 1 identifies the primary pharmacological target and mode of action, Axis 2 the approved indications, Axis 3 efficacy and side effects and Axis 4 human and animal neurobiology. NbNomenclature is available as a free downloadable app for Android phones and iPhones/iPads.

Although there is dissatisfaction with the current nomenclature, and a wish to apply pharmacological knowledge to clinical use of drugs, it remains to be seen whether this new system will pass into general use. Given that we still lack sufficient knowledge of the key mechanism/s of action of drugs used in psychiatry, and how their pharmacology relates to clinical action, the Axis 1 classification has to be viewed as provisional. In addition, the multi-axial system is somewhat cumbersome for clinical use. We have therefore decided not to adopt the NbNomenclature system for this book. For ease of use, we have retained the (admittedly imperfect) historic clinically based groupings of drugs, but detail their currently known pharmacology.

Ian M Anderson
R Hamish McAllister-Williams

List of abbreviations

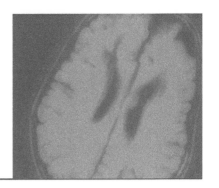

1-PP	1-(2-Pyrimidinyl)piperazine
2-AG	2-Arachidonylglycerol
5-HT	5-Hydroxytryptamine, serotonin
5-HTP	5-Hydroxytryptophan
5-HTPDC	5-HTP decarboxylase
5-HIAA	5-Hydroxyindoleacetic acid
5-HTT	5-HT transporter
5-HTTLPR	Serotonin transporter linked promoter polymorphism
AC	Adenylate cyclase
ACE	Angiotensin-converting enzyme
ACh	Acetylcholine
AChE	Acetylcholinesterase
AChEI	Acetylcholinesterase inhibitor
AD	Alzheimer's disease
ADAS-cog	Alzheimer's Disease Assessment Scale-cognitive subscale
ADH	Antidiuretic hormone
ADHD	Attention deficit/hyperactivity disorder
ADL	Activities of daily living
ALDH	Aldehyde dehydrogenase
AMP	Adenosine monophosphate
AMPA	Amino-3-hydroxy-5-methyl-isoxazole propionate
AMTS	Abbreviated Mental Test Score
AP5	2-Amino-5-phosphopentanoic acid
ApoE	Apolipoprotein E
APP	Amyloid precursor protein
ASD	Autism spectrum disorder
ATP	Adenosine triphosphate
ATPase	Adenosine triphosphatase
AUC	Area under the curve

β-CCE	Ethyl-β-carboline-3-carboxylate
BD	Bipolar disorder
BDI	Beck Depression Inventory
BDNF	Brain-derived neurotrophic factor
BDZ	Benzodiazepine
BEHAVE-AD	Behavioural Pathology in Alzheimer's Disease scale
BNF	British National Formulary
BPSD	Behavioural and psychiatric symptoms of dementia
Ca^{2+}	Calcium
cAMP	Cyclic adenosine monophosphate, cyclic AMP
CB	Cannabinoid
CBT	Cognitive behavioural therapy
CCK	Cholecystokinin
CCK4	Cholecystokinin tetrapeptide
CDR	Clinical Dementia Rating
ChAT	Choline acetyltransferase
CIBIC	Clinician Interview Based Impression of Change
Cl^-	Chloride
C_{max}	Maximum plasma concentration (pharmacokinetics)
CNS	Central nervous system
CO_2	Carbon dioxide
CoA	Coenzyme-A
COMT	Catechol-O-methyltransferase
COX-2	Cyclooxygenase-2
C_p	Plasma concentration (pharmacokinetics)
CRE	cAMP response elements
CREB	cAMP response element binding protein
CRF	Corticotrophin-releasing factor
CRP	C-reactive protein
CSF	Cerebrospinal fluid
CYP/CYP450	Cytochrome P450
D	Dopamine (used for receptor terminology)
DA	Dopamine
DAG	Diacylglycerol
DAT	Dopamine transporter
DβH	Dopamine-β-hydroxlase
DOPA	Dihydroxyphenylalanine
DOPAC	Dihydroxyphenylacetic acid
DOPADC	DOPA decarboxylase
DSM-IV/5	Fourth/fifth revision of the *Diagnostic and Statistical Manual of Mental Disease* (American Psychiatric Association)
EAAT	Excitatory amino acid transporters
ECG	Electrocardiogram

ECT	Electroconvulsive therapy
EEG	Electroencephalogram
EPSE	Extrapyramidal side effects
EU	European Union
FBC	Full blood count
FDA	Food and Drugs Administration (United States regulator)
FMO	Flavin-containing monooxygenase
G	Guanine nucleotide
GABA	γ (gamma) aminobutyric acid
GAD	Generalised anxiety disorder, glutamic acid decarboxylase
GBL	Gamma-butyrolactone
GCP	Good clinical practice
GDP	Guanosine diphosphate
GFR	Glomerular filtration rate
GHB	Gamma-hydroxybutyrate
GI	Gastrointestinal
G_i	Inhibitory G-protein
GIRK	G-protein-linked inward rectifying potassium channel
GluT	Glutamate transporter
GlyT	Glycine transporter
GPCR	G-protein-coupled receptor
G_s	Stimulatory G-protein
GTP	Guanosine triphosphate
GTPase	Guanosine triphosphatase
GSK-3β	Glycogen synthase kinase 3 beta
H	Histamine
HERG	Human ether-a-go-go (gene)
HLA	Human leucocyte antigen
HPA	Hypothalmic—pituitary—adrenal
HRT	Hormone replacement therapy
HVA	Homovanillic acid
IADL	Instrumental Activities of Daily Living
ICD-10	Tenth revision of the *International Classification of Diseases* (World Health Organisation)
IDDD	Interview for Deterioration in Daily Living in Dementia
I_{Kr}	Delayed rectifier K^+ channel
IL-6	Interleukin-6
im	Intramuscular
IP_3	Inositol trisphosphate
IPT	Interpersonal therapy
ITT	Intention to treat
iv	Intravenous
K^+	Potassium

LAAM	Levo-alpha-acetylmethadol
LAT1	L-type amino acid transporter 1
LC	Locus coeruleus
L-DOPA	L-dihydroxyphenylanine
LFTs	Liver function tests
LOCF	Last observation carried forward
LSD	Lysergic acid diethylamide
LTA	Lateral tegmental area
LTP	Long-term potentiation
mACh(R)	Muscarinic acetylcholine (receptor)
MAO	Monoamine oxidase
MAOI	Monoamine oxidase inhibitor
MAPK	Mitogen-activated protein kinase
MDA	Methylenedioxyamfetamine/ methylenedioxyamphetamine
MDD	Major depressive disorder
MDEA	Methylenedioxyethylamfetamine/ methylenedioxyethylamphetamine
MDMA	Methylenedioxymethamfetamine/ methylenedioxymethamphetamine
MDPV	3,4-Methylenedioxypyrovalerone
MEMO	Medicines Monitoring (Unit)
Mg^{2+}	Magnesium
mGLuR	Metabotropic glutamate receptor
MHPG	3-Methoxy-4-hydroxyphenylglycol
MHRA	Medicines and Healthcare Products Regulatory Authority (United Kingdom)
MK-801	Dizocilpine
MMRM	Mixed effects model repeated measures
MMSE	Mini-Mental State Examination
MPAC	Metal protein attenuating compound
M-PEM	Modified prescription event monitoring
MT	Methoxytyramine, melatonin
MTA	Multimodal Treatment Study of ADHD
NA	Noradrenaline (norepinephrine)
Na^+	Sodium
nACh(R)	Nicotinic acetylcholine (receptor)
NARI	Noradrenaline reuptake inhibitor
NaSSa	Noradrenaline- and serotonin-specific antidepressant
NAT	Noradrenaline transporter
NICE	National Institute for Health and Care Excellence (United Kingdom)
NK	Neurokinin
NM	Normetanephrine

NMDA	*N*-methyl D-aspartate
NMS	Neuroleptic malignant syndrome
NPI	Neuropsychiatric Inventory
NPY	Neuropeptide Y
NSAID	Nonsteroidal anti-inflammatory drug
NT	Neurotensin
OCD	Obsessive-compulsive disorder
OPCS	Office of Population Censuses and Surveys
OR	Odds ratio
OX	Orexin
PAG	Periaqueductal grey
PCB	Polychlorinated biphenyl
PCP	Phencyclidine
PEM	Prescription event monitoring
PET	Positron emission tomography
PHQ-9	Patient Health Questionnaire-9
PLC	Phospholipase-C
PNMT	Phenylethanolamine-N-methyltransferase
PPARγ	Peroxisome proliferator-activated receptor gamma
PPI	Patient and public involvement
PROM	Patient reported outcome measure
PTSD	Post-traumatic stress disorder
Q	Quantity of drug (pharmacokinetics)
QTc	Interval between Q and T waves on the electrocardiogram corrected for heart rate
RCT	Randomised controlled trial
REM	Rapid eye movement
RIMA	Reversible inhibitor of monoamine oxidase-A
RTK	Receptor tyrosine kinase
SCEM	Specialised cohort event monitoring
SERT	Serotonin (5-HT) transporter
SIADH	Syndrome of inappropriate ADH secretion
SJS	Stevens–Johnson syndrome
SMARTS	Systematic Monitoring of Adverse Events Related to Treatments
SmPC	Summary of product characteristics
SNAP-25	Synaptosomal-associated protein 25
SNRI	Serotonin and noradrenaline reuptake inhibitor
SPECT	Single photon emission computerised tomography
SSRI	Selective serotonin reuptake inhibitor
SUCRA	Surface under the cumulative response curve

$t\frac{1}{2}$	Half-life (pharmacokinetics)
T3	Triiodothyronine
TCA	Tricyclic antidepressant
TH	Tyrosine hydroxylase
THA	Tacrine, tetrahydroaminoacridine
THC	δ-9-Tetrahydrocannabinol
t_{max}	Time to maximum (peak) plasma concentration
TNFα	Tumour necrosis factor-α
TPH	Tryptophan hydroxylase
TRH	Thyrotropin-releasing hormone
TRK-B	Tropomyosin receptor kinase B
TSH	Thyroid-stimulating hormone
UK	United Kingdom
US/USA	United States/United States of America
V_d	Volume of distribution (pharmacokinetics)
VGAT	Vesicular GABA transporter (also VIAAT)
VGLUT	Vesicular glutamate transporter
VIAAT	Vesicular inhibitory amino acid transporter (also VGAT)
VMAT	Vesicular monoamine transporter
VNTR	Variable number tandem repeat
VTA	Ventral tegmental area
Zn^{2+}	Zinc

Contributors

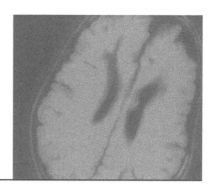

Ian M Anderson
Neuroscience and Psychiatry Unit
The University of Manchester
Manchester, United Kingdom

David S Baldwin
Department of Psychiatry
University of Southampton
Southampton, United Kingdom

Frances Cheng
Department of Psychiatry
The University of Hong Kong
Pokfulam, Hong Kong

David R Coghill
Division of Neuroscience
University of Dundee
Dundee, United Kingdom

Mark Daglish
Hospital Alcohol and Drug Service
Royal Brisbane & Women's
Hospital
Brisbane, Queensland, Australia

Sarah E Gartside
Institute of Neuroscience
Newcastle University
Newcastle upon Tyne,
United Kingdom

Peter M Haddad
Department of Psychiatry
Greater Manchester West Mental
Health NHS Foundation Trust
and
The University of Manchester
Salford, United Kingdom

Mehran Javeed
Department of Old Age Psychiatry
Manchester Mental Health and
Social Care NHS Trust
Manchester, United Kingdom

Peter B Jones
Department of Psychiatry
University of Cambridge
Cambridge, United Kingdom

Stephen M Lawrie
Division of Psychiatry
The University of Edinburgh
Edinburgh, United Kingdom

Iracema Leroi
Institute of Brain, Behaviour and
Mental Health
The University of Manchester
Manchester, United Kingdom

Anne Lingford-Hughes
Centre for Neuropsycho-
pharmacology
Imperial College London
London, United Kingdom

Charles A Marsden
School of Life Sciences
University of Nottingham
Nottingham, United Kingdom

R Hamish McAllister-Williams
Institute of Neuroscience
Newcastle University
Newcastle upon Tyne,
United Kingdom

Chris Smart
Institute of Neuroscience
Newcastle University
Newcastle upon Tyne,
United Kingdom

Peter S Talbot
Wolfson Molecular Imaging Centre
The University of Manchester
Manchester, United Kingdom

Nupur Tiwari
Department of Psychiatry
University of Southampton
Southampton, United Kingdom

Birgit A Völlm
Institute of Mental Health
University of Nottingham
Nottingham, United Kingdom

Angelika Wieck
Department of Psychiatry
Manchester Mental Health and
Social Care NHS Trust
and
The University of Manchester
Manchester, United Kingdom

Sarah C Wooderson
Centre for Affective Disorders
King's College London
London, United Kingdom

Allan H Young
Centre for Affective Disorders
King's College London
London, United Kingdom

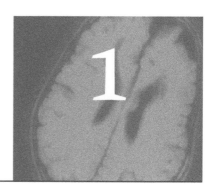

Neuropharmacology and drug action

Sarah E Gartside and Charles A Marsden

 ## Introduction

This chapter will concentrate on neurotransmission and the mechanisms by which psychotropic drugs alter neurotransmission.

- Most drugs used in psychiatry, as well as non-therapeutic psychotropic drugs, act to alter neurotransmission.
- In general, drugs act either *presynaptically* to influence levels of the neurotransmitter in the synaptic cleft, or *postsynaptically* by agonist, antagonist or modulatory actions at postsynaptic receptors.

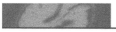 ## Neurotransmission

- Neurotransmission describes the process by which information is transferred from one neuron to another neuron (or other cell type) across the synaptic cleft (Figure 1.1). It involves
  - The release of a neurotransmitter from the presynaptic nerve ending in response to the arrival of an action potential
  - The subsequent activation of a receptor on the membrane of the postsynaptic neuron
- Activation of the postsynaptic receptor may result either in
  - *Excitation* – membrane depolarisation
  - *Inhibition* – membrane hyperpolarisation
- These membrane effects may be due to either
  - A direct effect on an ion channel (*fast neurotransmission*; Figure 1.2), or
  - An indirect effect via a guanine nucleotide–binding (G) protein to cause the opening of ion channels, or the stimulation or inhibition of an enzyme and consequent increase or decrease in a second messenger (*slow neurotransmission*; Figure 1.2) (see Section Receptor mechanisms)

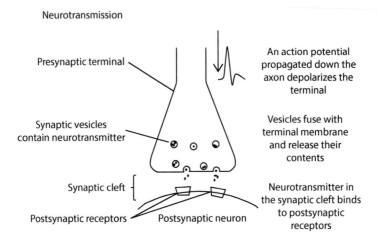

Figure 1.1 Synaptic transmission involves release of a neurotransmitter from the presynaptic nerve ending and its binding to a postsynaptic receptor to produce a change in function (excitation or inhibition) in the postsynaptic neuron.

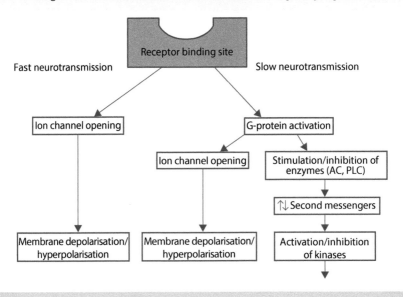

Figure 1.2 Fast neurotransmission is mediated by ligand-gated ion channel receptors (e.g. glutamate NMDA and $GABA_A$ receptors) and involves direct opening of an ion channel. Slow neurotransmission is mediated through G-protein-coupled receptors (e.g. D_2 receptors and $5\text{-}HT_{1A}$ receptors) and involves indirect ion channel opening or production/inhibition of second messengers through action on adenlyate cyclase (AC) or phospholipase-C (PLC). Activation/inhibition of kinase enzymes by the second messengers cyclic adenosine monophosphate (cAMP) and diacylglycerol (DAG) leads to changes in intracellular processes including ion transport and enzyme activity.

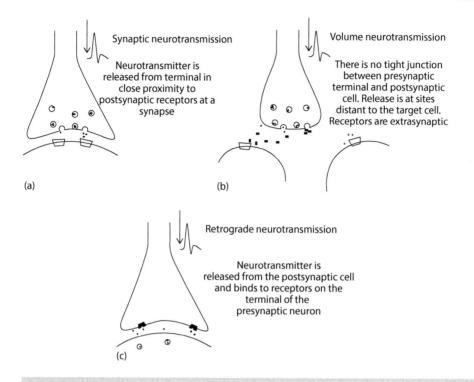

Figure 1.3 Different modalities of neurotransmission/signalling. (a) Synaptic transmission is rapid and point-to-point, transmission from presynaptic terminal to postsynaptic cell. (b) Volume transmission is slower, involves release of neurotransmitter at a distance from its target sites which are extrasynaptic receptors. (c) Retrograde signalling involves the activity-dependent release of a substance from the postsynaptic cell which then affects release of transmitter from the presynaptic terminal.

▓ Originally, all neurotransmissions were considered to be *synaptic* (i.e. rapid, point-to-point, from presynaptic terminal to postsynaptic cell). However, there is now evidence for other mechanisms (see Figure 1.3) including

– *Extrasynaptic volume transmission* involves the release of neurotransmitter at a distance from its target, extrasynaptic receptor, sites. This is slower than synaptic transmission, and believed to underlie the modulatory and tuning functions of many neurotransmitters (e.g. monoamines and nitric oxide).

– *Retrograde signalling* involves the activity-dependent release of a substance from the postsynaptic cell which then affects release of transmitter from the presynaptic terminal (e.g. endocannabinoid modulation of glutamate and GABA neurotransmission).

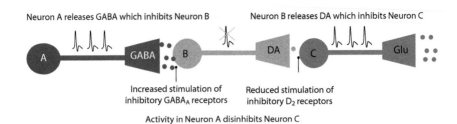

Neuron A releases GABA which inhibits Neuron B   Neuron B releases DA which inhibits Neuron C

Increased stimulation of inhibitory $GABA_A$ receptors   Reduced stimulation of inhibitory D_2 receptors

Activity in Neuron A disinhibits Neuron C

Figure 1.4 The initial receptor response (i.e. excitation or inhibition) does not necessarily describe the final functional output. In this example, increased activity in an inhibitory neuron (Neuron A) ultimately causes disinhibition (excitation) of a downstream neuron (Neuron C). The net response is excitation.

- The initial receptor response (i.e. excitation or inhibition) does not necessarily describe the final functional output: For example inhibition of an inhibitory neuron will cause disinhibition of the next neuron in the chain and thus a net excitatory response (see Figure 1.4). Behaviour is thus the result of a complex interplay between many neurons, and it is very difficult to explain a particular behaviour as being the result of the action of a single neurotransmitter.

Co-existence of neurotransmitters

- The major neurotransmitters in the brain are *noradrenaline* (NA, also called norepinephrine), *dopamine* (DA), *5-hydroxytryptamine* (5-HT, also called serotonin), *acetylcholine* (ACh), *glutamate* and *γ-aminobutyric acid* (GABA). Neurons are described with respect to the neurotransmitter they synthesize and release (e.g. dopaminergic, serotonergic, GABAergic).
- The original concept of chemical neurotransmission posited that only one active substance (neurotransmitter) was released from the presynaptic terminal, but we now know that two or more biologically active substances are often released in response to an action potential.
- DA, NA, 5-HT and ACh commonly co-exist with various neuropeptides, for example cholecystokinin (CCK), neurotensin (NT), thyrotrophin-releasing hormone (TRH) and orexin (also known as hypocretin) which act as either.
  - *Full neurotransmitters* (i.e. produce a functional response on their own)
  - *Neuromodulators* (i.e. they modulate the response to the main neurotransmitter)
- Coexistence is probably the normal state of affairs, although its functional importance, and potential impact on drug treatment, is poorly understood.

- Neurohypophysial hormones (e.g. corticotrophin releasing factor [CRF] and oxytocin) also act as neuromodulators within the brain in addition to their hormonal actions.

Overview of neurotransmitters

Table 1.1 lists the major neurotransmitters in the brain together with the functions and neurological/psychiatric disorders in which they are thought to play a role.

Table 1.1 Central nervous system neurotransmitters and neuromodulators

Class	Neurotransmitter	Function/disorder
Amines	Acetylcholine (ACh)	Alzheimer's disease
	Dopamine (DA)	Parkinson's disease, schizophrenia, depression
	Noradrenaline (NA)	Anxiety, depression, cognition, schizophrenia
	5-Hydroxytryptamine (serotonin, 5-HT)	Depression, anxiety/panic/OCD, schizophrenia, Alzheimer's disease, migraine, hallucinations, eating disorders
	Histamine	Arousal, cognition
Amino acids	Glutamate	Neurodegeneration, schizophrenia, depression
	γ-Aminobutyric acid (GABA)	Anxiety, Huntington's disease
Peptides	Met/leu-enkephalin	Pain, mood
	β-Endorphin	Pain, mood
	Substance P/tachykinins	Huntington's disease, depression
	Vasopressin	Cognition
	Cholecystokinin (CCK)	Anxiety, pain
	Somatostatin	Mood
	Neurotensin (NT)	Schizophrenia
	Thyrotropin-releasing hormone (TRH)	Arousal, motor neuron disease
	Neuropeptide Y (NPY)	Feeding
	Corticotrophin-releasing factor (CRF)	Anxiety, depression
	Orexins	Circadian function, feeding, response to stress
Other	Endocannabinoids	Pain, schizophrenia, eating disorders

Note: The major neurotransmitters and neuromodulators together with the functions and disorders with which they are associated.

In addition to the neurotransmitters mentioned earlier, many other chemicals are now known to act as neurotransmitters or neuromodulators in the brain.

- The *enkephalins* (leu-enkephalin and met-enkephalin) along with β-endorphin and the dynorphins are closely structurally related peptides acting as endogenous ligands for the mu (μ), delta (δ) and kappa (κ) opioid receptors and are widely distributed in the brain. They have important roles in pain, addictive behaviours and emotional responding.
- The *neurokinins* substance P (neurokinin-1), substance K (neurokinin-2 or neurokinin A) and neuromedin K (neurokinin B) are a group of peptides which act on NK_1, NK_2 and NK_3 receptors. They have a role as neurotransmitters and neuromodulators and are involved in inflammation. Antagonists of NK_1 and NK_3 receptors have been investigated in the treatment of depression, schizophrenia and neurodegenerative disorders.
- *Neurotensin* (NT) is a peptide which acts on neurotensin receptors (NT1–4) and is present in the amygdala and in basal forebrain and brainstem nuclei. NT is co-localised with DA in the ventral tegmental area and has been shown to modify DAergic neurotransmission. NT has been implicated in schizophrenia and addictive behaviours.
- *Cholecystokinins* (CCKs) are a family of neuropeptides which are particularly concentrated in the amygdala and periaqueductal grey (PAG) as well as other brain regions implicated in fear and anxiety. In the brain, the actions of CCKs are mediated by CCK2 (or CCKB) receptors. Although the tetrapeptide of CCK, CCK4, induces panic attacks, CCK receptor antagonists are ineffective as antipanic drugs, possibly related to poor brain penetration of the compounds.
- *Corticotrophin-releasing factor* (CRF) acts on CRF_1 and CRF_2 receptors in the pituitary gland (leading to the secretion of ACTH and cortisol) and other brain areas such as the amygdala, locus coeruleus (LC) and hippocampus. CRF is involved in the stress response and has mood and cognitive effects. CRF_1 antagonists are being evaluated as antidepressants, anxiolytics and as a treatment for alcohol dependence.
- *Somatostatin* is a peptide hormone that acts on G-protein-coupled somatostatin receptors. It inhibits release of growth hormone and thyroid-stimulating hormone from the anterior pituitary. It also acts as a modulator of neurotransmission and cell proliferation. It has been implicated in the pathophysiology of mood disorders.
- *Orexins A* and *B* (hypocretins) are closely related neuropeptides derived from a single gene. They act on OX_1 and OX_2 receptors which are highly expressed in the lateral hypothalamus and other brain areas involved in stress regulation. Orexins were initially identified as important regulators of feeding, but are also involved in circadian function, sleep and response to stress including neuroendocrine control.

- The *endocannabinoids*, which include anandamide, are the endogenous agonists of cannabinoid type 1 (CB_1) and type 2 (CB_2) receptors. Brain CB_1 receptors regulate the release of glutamate and GABA through retrograde neurotransmission (see Figure 1.4). CB_1 receptors are potential targets for the treatment of pain and mood disorders. CB_2 receptors are associated with the immune system.
- *Neuroactive steroids* (steroids synthesised, and/or are active, in the brain) interact with nuclear steroid receptors, and have also been shown to modulate the function of $GABA_A$ receptors both positively and negatively. They have been implicated in the pathogenesis of anxiety, cognitive and affective disorders. Drugs interacting with the neurosteroid system are potential anxiolytics.
- *Brain-derived neurotrophic factor* (BDNF) is one of several neurotrophic factors which have important roles in the normal development of the brain as well as in maintaining synaptic function and mediating synaptic plasticity in the adult brain. BDNF, which acts on TRK-B (tropomyosin receptor kinase B) receptors, has been shown to be increased by chronic treatment with antidepressant drugs and non-drug therapies in animals, and hence has been postulated to be involved in their therapeutic mechanism of action.

Organisation of neurotransmitter pathways

The major neurotransmitter pathways – and those most important in psychopharmacology – can be divided organisationally into three groups:

- *Long ascending and descending axonal pathways* derived from discrete neuronal cell groups located within specific brain nuclei. This organisation is a feature of catecholaminergic (DA, NA), serotonergic (5-HT) and histaminergic (HA), as well as many cholinergic (ACh), pathways (see Figure 1.5).
- *Long and short axonal pathways* derived from neuronal cell bodies widely distributed throughout the brain. Neurons which contain the major excitatory (glutamate) and inhibitory (GABA) neurotransmitters are organised in this way.
- *Short intraregional pathways* within the cerebral cortex, striatum, etc. Many of these so-called 'interneurons' are GABAergic, but various neuropeptidergic neurons (e.g. somatostatin neurons in the cerebral cortex) are organised in this way.

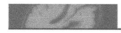 ## Receptor mechanisms

The main targets for current psychotropic drug action are receptors and transporters.

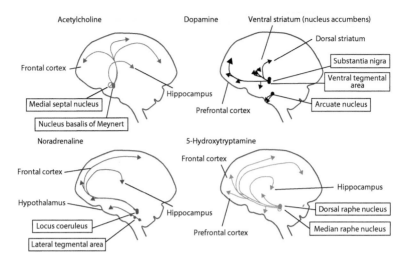

Figure 1.5 The main pathways in the brain of cholinergic, dopaminergic, noradrenergic and serotonergic neurons. Note the discrete localisation of the neuronal cell bodies and the long ascending projections.

- Receptors for neurotransmitters are mostly located on the *cell membrane*. Neurotransmitters or drugs acting on the receptor bind to an external domain, resulting in a response within the neuron. There are two main types of neurotransmitter receptor:
  - *Ligand-gated ion channel* (or ionotropic*)* receptors are directly coupled to an ion channel and mediate fast neurotransmission. Examples include *N*-methyl-D-aspartate (NMDA) (glutamate) receptors, GABA$_A$ receptors and nicotinic ACh (nACh) receptors.
  - *G-protein-coupled* (or metabotropic) receptors link the binding of the ligand to an intracellular effector system via a G-protein. These receptors mediate slow neurotransmission. Examples include DA D$_1$ and D$_2$ receptors, α- and β-adrenoceptors, most 5-HT receptors and muscarinic ACh (mACh) receptors.
- Additional types of receptors include
  - *Intracellular steroid receptors* (e.g. glucocorticoid receptors). These reside in the cytosol of cells, and when bound by ligand, they translocate to the cell nucleus where they bind to DNA, influencing transcription. Abnormalities in the function of these receptors have been implicated in psychiatric disorders including anxiety and mood disorders
  - *Receptor tyrosine kinases* (RTKs) are cell surface receptors for many peptide growth factors and cytokines. They are of increasing interest in psychiatry due to findings of raised pro-inflammatory cytokines in many conditions including schizophrenia and depression

Ligand-gated ion channel receptors

- Ligand-gated ion channel receptors consist of four (tetramer) or five (pentamer) protein subunits arranged to form a central channel or pore.
- Binding of the neurotransmitter (or other agonist) to the receptor causes a conformational (shape) change in the proteins which results in the opening of the channel, allowing specific ions to pass through.
- Ion channels open within milliseconds and allow the passage of ions through the cell membrane, leading to rapid excitatory or inhibitory effects on the cell.
- Excitatory ligand-gated ion channels (e.g. glutamate NMDA and AMPA receptors, nACh receptors) are permeable to sodium ions (Na^+) (and in some cases calcium ions, Ca^{2+}) which flow into the cell, causing membrane depolarisation. The inhibitory ligand-gated ion channels (e.g. $GABA_A$ receptors) are permeable to chloride ions (Cl^-) which enter the cell, causing hyperpolarisation.

G-protein-coupled receptors (Figure 1.6)

- G-proteins provide the link between the ligand recognition site and the effector system, and are so named because their action is linked to effects on an associated *guanine nucleotide–binding* (G) *protein*.
- G-protein-coupled receptors (GPCRs) consist of a single protein which crosses the cell membrane seven times, with loops inside and outside of the cell. The ligand (neurotransmitter or drug) binds to external parts of the protein. One of the internal loops, which is larger than the rest, interacts with the G-protein.
- The G-protein has three subunits (α, β, γ). The α subunit contains *guanosine triphosphatase* (GTPase) activity.
- When the transmitter or other agonist binds to the receptor, α-*guanosine triphosphate* (α-GTP) is released, which then can either activate or inhibit one of the two major second messenger systems:
  - *Cyclic adenosine monophosphate* (cAMP), produced by the enzyme *adenylate cyclase* (also called adenylyl cyclase), activates protein kinases, which in turn influence the function of various enzymes, carriers, etc. Receptors can be either positively or negatively coupled to adenylate cyclase, causing stimulation (*excitation*) or *inhibition* of the enzyme, respectively (Figure 1.6)
  - *Phospholipase C–inositol trisphosphate* (IP_3)–*diacylglycerol* (DAG) system: Activation of the enzyme *phospholipase C* results in the formation of two intracellular messengers, IP_3 and DAG. IP_3 increases free calcium (Ca^{2+}) which activates various enzymes. DAG activates *protein kinase C*, which in turn regulates various intracellular functions

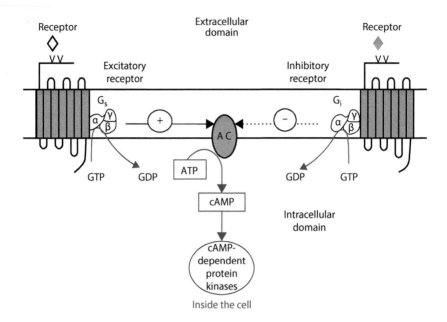

Figure 1.6   G-proteins couple the receptor binding site to the second messenger system, and they consist of three subunits (α, β, γ) anchored to the seven trans-membrane helices that form the receptor. Coupling of the α-subunit to an ago-nist-occupied receptor causes bound guanine diphosphate (GDP) to exchange with guanine triphosphate (GTP) and the resulting α-GTP complex leaves the receptor to interact with a target protein (an enzyme such as adenylate cyclase [AC] or an ion channel). There is then hydrolysis of the bound GTP to GDP, and the α subunit links again to the $\beta\gamma$ subunit. The G-protein mechanism can be either inhibitory (G_i) or excitatory (G_s).

> G-proteins can also be linked to potassium (K^+) and Ca^{2+} channels and so regulate membrane excitability and transmitter release: For example the 5-HT_{1A} cell body autoreceptor opens a K^+ channel, caus-ing hyperpolarisation, while activation of the 5-HT_{1B} terminal auto-receptor blocks Ca^{2+} channels, reducing neurotransmitter release.

Downstream signalling cascades

Although most drugs act initially through modification of neurotransmis-sion, many have long-term *neuroadaptive effects* due to actions *downstream* from the immediate postsynaptic mechanisms.

> These include changes in the expression of genes encoding growth fac-tors, including BDNF, vascular endothelial growth factor and fibroblast

growth factor-2, which are important in neuronal plasticity and long-term memory.

- Drug-induced changes in gene expression (e.g. of BDNF) often occur as a result of altered expression of the transcription factor family *CREB* (cAMP response element–binding protein), which binds in turn to DNA sequences called *cAMP response elements* (CREs).
- These effects underlie the *neurotrophic and neuroplasticity* hypothesis of antidepressant drug action (see Chapter 4).
- Drug treatment may also result in *epigenetic effects* (regulation of DNA transcription by mechanisms such as reduced DNA methylation and histone deacetylation), which are partly driven by changes in the expression of growth factors such as BDNF.

Receptor location

The location of a receptor determines its effects on neurotransmission (Figure 1.7).

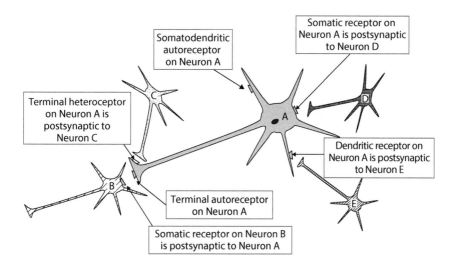

Figure 1.7 The nomenclature used to describe receptor location on neurons. Starting with 'Neuron A', neurotransmitter released at the terminals will interact with postsynaptic receptors on 'Neuron B'. Similarly, neurotransmitter released from 'Neurons D and E' will interact with postsynaptic receptor on 'Neuron A'. Neurotransmitter released from 'Neuron A' will also regulate its own release by interacting with the terminal autoreceptor or affect neuronal firing by interacting with the somatodendritic autoreceptor. Release of neurotransmitter from 'Neuron A' can also be regulated by activation of presynaptic heteroceptors on the terminals which are postsynaptic receptors activated by neurotransmitter from 'Neuron C'.

- Receptors are mostly located on a membrane on the far side of the synaptic cleft to the point of neurotransmitter release. These so-called *postsynaptic receptors* may be located on
  - Dendrites or the soma (cell body) of a neuron where they regulate cell firing. An example of this is nACh receptors on the cell bodies of DAergic neurons in the ventral tegmental area.
  - Nerve terminals where they regulate neurotransmitter release (sometimes referred to as *presynaptic heteroceptors*). An example of this is the presence of inhibitory α_2-adrenoceptors on the terminals of 5-HT neurons.
- Receptors located on the same type of neuron that releases the neurotransmitter that activates it are termed *autoreceptors* and are concerned with autoregulation (normally inhibitory feedback). Autoreceptors located on the soma or dendrites of the neuron (*somatodendritic autoreceptors*) regulate neuronal firing. Autoreceptors located on the presynaptic terminal (*terminal autoreceptors*) regulate neurotransmitter release.
- For most neurons, the same receptor subtype functions as the somatodendritic and terminal autoreceptor. Thus, D_2, α_2 and mACh receptors are both somatodendritic and terminal autoreceptors for DAergic, NAergic and cholinergic neurons, respectively. In the case of 5-HT neurons, the somatodendritic autoreceptor is of the 5-HT$_{1A}$ subtype, whilst the terminal autoreceptors are of the 5-HT$_{1B}$ or 5-HT$_{1D}$ subtypes.
- In addition to terminal autoreceptors and heteroceptors, the release of neurotransmitter from the nerve terminal can also be inhibited by endocannabinoids through retrograde signalling (see Figure 1.3c).

Neurotransmitter transporters

Transporters are a second major target for psychotropic drugs:

- Most neurotransmitters are removed from the synaptic cleft by *high-affinity transporters*.
- This process limits the concentration and duration of neurotransmitter in the synaptic cleft, and so influences the action of a neurotransmitter on postsynaptic and presynaptic receptors.
- Neurotransmitter transporters:
  - They are a family of single protein chains which cross the neuronal membrane 12 times.
  - They co-transport Na^+ ions into the cell, with the Na^+ concentration gradient driving the movement of the neurotransmitter. This co-transport makes neurotransmitter transporters electrogenic (i.e. they cause current to flow across the membrane).

- Many antidepressant drugs (e.g. tricyclic antidepressants, selective serotonin reuptake inhibitors [SSRIs], noradrenaline reuptake inhibitors [NARIs]) block monoamine transporters.
  - The high sequence homology between transporters for DA (DAT), NA (NAT) and 5-HT (SERT or 5-HTT) means that many drugs have poor selectivity between transporters (e.g. most tricyclic antidepressants block both 5-HTT and NAT).
  - Inside the nerve terminal, monoamine neurotransmitters are moved from the cytosol into the storage vesicles by a protein transporter which is embedded in the vesicular membrane. All monoamine neurons contain the same vesicular transporter called *vesicular monoamine transporter-2* (VMAT2).
  - Drugs which belong to the amphetamine (amfetamine) class gain entry to nerve terminals via the membrane transporter (DAT, NAT and/or SERT). Once inside the terminal, they interact with VMAT2 to cause the release of the neurotransmitter independently of cell firing and terminal membrane depolarisation. The neurotransmitter selectivity of the various amphetamine derivatives, e.g. methylenedioxymethamphetamine (MDMA, ecstasy) (affecting 5-HT, NA and DA), methamphetamine (DA) and fenfluramine (5-HT), is determined by their affinity for the particular membrane transporter.
- There are four known types of GABA transporter with different structure, distribution and pharmacology. Inhibitors of GABA transport (e.g. tiagabine) have anticonvulsant activity.
- *Vesicular glutamate transporters* (VGlut1, 2 and 3) are found on both the plasma and vesicular membranes. Inhibitors of glutamate transport currently have no therapeutic use.

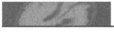 Individual neurotransmitters

Dopamine

Pathways and functions

DA-containing neuronal cell bodies are located in three discrete areas (Figure 1.5):

- *Substantia nigra* – Axons project from this midbrain area to the basal ganglia (dorsal striatum, caudate-putamen).
  - They are involved in the initiation of motor plans and motor co-ordination.
  - This pathway is the primary site of degeneration in Parkinson's disease.
  - Antipsychotic drugs (D_2-receptor antagonists) produce motor disturbances by blocking D_2 receptors in the caudate-putamen.

- *Ventral tegmental area* (VTA) – Axons project to the nucleus accumbens (ventral striatum) and amygdala, and to the prefrontal cortex. These are referred to as the *mesolimbic* and *mesocortical* DA pathways, respectively. These pathways are strongly associated with motivation, reward behaviour and drug dependence as well as with cognition. Many drugs of abuse increase DA transmission in these pathways, e.g. amphetamines cause DA release, cocaine blocks DA re-uptake, while opioids and cannabinoids (disinhibition) and nicotine, all increase the firing of DA neurons (see Chapter 7). These pathways are also considered important in schizophrenia and are an important site of action for antipsychotic drugs (D_2 and D_4 antagonists).
- *Tuberoinfundibular DA pathway* – Neurons in the median eminence project to the pituitary. In the anterior pituitary, DA released from the median eminence inhibits prolactin release via activation of D_2 receptors. Drugs that block D_2 receptors (e.g. antipsychotics) increase (disinhibit) prolactin secretion which accounts for the side effects of gynaecomastia, galactorrhoea and amenorrhoea, frequently observed with antipsychotic drugs.

Synthesis and metabolism (Table 1.2, Figure 1.8)

- DA is synthesised from the amino acid tyrosine, by the actions of the enzymes tyrosine hydroxylase and DOPA decarboxylase. L-Tyrosine is first hydroxylated to form the intermediate L-dihydroxyphenylalanine (L-DOPA) which is in turn decarboxylated to form DA (Table 1.2). Tyrosine hydroxylase, the rate-limiting enzyme in this synthetic pathway, is inhibited by α-methyl-*para*-tyrosine.
- DA is stored in vesicles where it is protected from the degradation by monoamine oxidase (MAO).
- Following release, DA is taken back up into the presynaptic terminal by the DA transporter (DAT).
- DA is metabolised by mitochondrial MAO (isoforms A and B) and by the membrane-bound catechol-*O*-methyltransferase (COMT) enzyme to form homovanillic acid (HVA) (Table 1.2).
- Inhibitors of both MAO-B and COMT are used in the symptomatic treatment of Parkinson's disease.
- DA release is under inhibitory autoreceptor feedback regulation by the presynaptic D_2 and/or D_3 dopamine receptor. Activation of these receptors results in the inhibition of DA release.

DA receptors (Table 1.3)

- Five DA receptors have been identified using pharmacological and molecular biological methods. All are G-protein coupled.

Table 1.2 Neurotransmitter synthesis and metabolism

Transmitter	Precursor	Synthetic enzymes	Inactivation
Acetylcholine (ACh)	Choline Acetyl Co-A	ChAT	Extracellular AChE Choline taken up and recycled
Dopamine (DA)	Tyrosine	TH (to DOPA) DOPADC (to DA)	Reuptake followed by metabolism by MAO-A/B, and COMT
Noradrenaline (NA)	Tyrosine	TH (to DOPA) DOPADC (to DA) DβH (to NA)	Reuptake followed by metabolism by MAO-A and COMT
Serotonin (5-HT)	Tryptophan	TPH (to 5-HTP) 5-HTPDC (to 5-HT)	Reuptake followed by metabolism by MAO-A
Glutamate	Glutamine	Glutaminase	Reuptake followed by metabolism by GAD (GABA shunt)
GABA	Glutamate	GAD	Reuptake followed by metabolism by GABA-T

Note: Summary of the enzymes involved in the synthesis and metabolism of amine and amino acid neurotransmitters.

Key to abbreviations: AChE, acetylcholinesterase; ChAT, choline acetyltransferase; COMT, catechol-O-methyltransferase; DβH, dopamine-β-hydroxlase; DA, dopamine; DOPA, dihydroxyphenylalanine; DOPADC, DOPA decarboxylase; GABA-T, GABA transaminase; GAD, glutamic acid decarboxylase; 5-HTP, 5-hydroxytryptophan; 5-HTPDC, 5-HTP decarboxylase; MAO, monoamine oxidase; PNMT, phenylethanolamine-N-methyltransferase; TH, tyrosine hydroxylase; TPH, tryptophan hydroxylase.

- There are two families: The D_1-like comprising D_1 and D_5 receptors, which are positively coupled to adenylate cyclase, and the D_2-like (D_2, D_3, D_4) which are negatively coupled to adenylate cyclase.
- There are further variants, with short and long forms of the D_2 receptor, and genetic polymorphisms (D_4 in particular).
- Both D_1 and D_2 receptors have wide distribution (striatal, mesolimbic and hypothalamic regions), while D_3 and D_4 have a more restricted distribution (Table 1.3).
- The D_2 receptor is found both on DA neurons (as somatodendritic and terminal autoreceptor) and at postsynaptic sites. Thus, D_2 antagonists

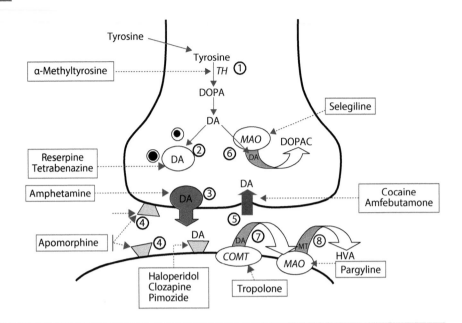

Figure 1.8 Schematic of a central dopaminergic terminal indicating possible sites of drug action. Tyrosine hydroxylase activity, and hence DA synthesis, is blocked by the irreversible competitive inhibitor, α-methyltyrosine (1). Reserpine and tetrabenazine interfere with the uptake-storage mechanism, causing damage to vesicles and long-lasting depletion of DA. The effects of reserpine are irreversible, while those of tetrabenazine do not appear to be irreversible (2). Amphetamine enters the terminal via the dopamine reuptake transporter DAT (5) and releases DA from the vesicles (3). Apomorphine is a non-selective DA receptor agonist with both pre- and postsynaptic sites of action. Haloperidol, pimozide, clozapine and other antipsychotics are D_2 receptor antagonists (4). Released DA has its action terminated by reuptake into presynaptic terminal. Cocaine and amfebutamone (bupropion) are inhibitors of this reuptake mechanism (5). DA present in the cytosol of the presynaptic terminal can be degraded by the enzyme monoamine oxidase (MAO) which is located in the outer membrane of the mitochondria (6). Dihydroxyphenylacetic acid (DOPAC) is a product of the action of MAO and aldehyde reductase on DA. Selegiline is an inhibitor of MAO-B. DA can also be inactivated to methoxytyramine (MT) by the enzyme catechol-O-methyl transferase (COMT), which is believed to be localised outside the presynaptic neuron. Tropolone is an inhibitor of COMT (7). Some MAO is also present outside the dopaminergic neuron (8) where it metabolises MT to HVA.

not only block postsynaptic responses but also increase DA release by blockade of autoreceptors.

■ Both typical and atypical antipsychotics have high affinity for D_2 receptors. However, atypical antipsychotics have lower affinity for D_2 receptors than typical antipsychotics which may contribute to their superior side-effect profile (see Chapter 3). The atypical antipsychotic clozapine has high affinity for the D_4 receptor which may be important in its distinct clinical profile.

Table 1.3 Dopamine receptors

| Distribution | Functional role | D$_1$-like | | D$_2$-like* | | |
		D$_1$	D$_5$	D$_2$	D$_3$	D$_4$
Cortex	Arousal, mood	++	—	++	—	—
Limbic system	Emotion, stereotypic behaviour	+++	—	+++	+	++
Basal ganglia	Motor control	++	+	+++	+	+
Hypothalamus	Autonomic and endocrine control	++	+	—	—	—
Pituitary gland	Endocrine control	—	—	+++	—	—
Signal transduction		Increase cAMP		Decrease cAMP		
Agonists	Dopamine	+ (low potency)		+ (high potency)		
	Bromocriptine	Partial agonist				
Antagonists	Chlorpromazine	+	+	+++	+++	+
	Haloperidol	++	+	+++	+++	+++
	Clozapine	+	+	+	+	++
Effect		Postsynaptic inhibition		Pre- and post-synaptic inhibition		

Note: The distribution, function, signal transduction and pharmacology of dopamine receptors in brain.
cAMP, cyclic adenosine monophosphate; —, not functionally involved; +, ++, +++, slightly, moderately, very, functionally involved, respectively; *, there are short and long forms of D$_2$ receptors and variants of D$_3$ and D$_4$.

Noradrenaline

Pathways and functions (Figure 1.5)

▪ The principal location of the cell bodies of NA-containing neurons is the locus coeruleus (LC) in the pons. Noradrenergic axons project up to limbic areas (via the *dorsal noradrenergic bundle*) and down to the spinal cord (involved in muscle co-ordination). Nuclei in the lateral tegmental area (LTA) of the medulla also contain noradrenergic cell bodies. Projections from the LTA innervate forebrain regions via the *ventral noradrenergic bundle*.

▪ LC and LTA neurons project to the hypothalamus, cortex and subcortical limbic areas.

▦ The cortical projections are concerned with arousal and maintaining the cortex in an alert state. The limbic projections are involved in drive, motivation, mood and response to stress.

Synthesis and metabolism (Table 1.2, Figure 1.9)

▦ NA is synthesised from tyrosine by the enzymes tyrosine hydroxylase and DOPA decarboxylase (see Section DA receptors). The resulting DA is converted to NA by the action of a third enzyme, dopamine-β-hydroxylase (Table 1.2), which is found exclusively in noradrenergic and adrenergic neurons.

▦ NA is stored in vesicles protected from MAO and ready for release in response to terminal depolarisation.

▦ The action of released NA on receptors is terminated by reuptake via NAT; a process inhibited by tricyclic antidepressants, reboxetine, venlafaxine and duloxetine as well as cocaine.

▦ NA, like DA, is metabolised by MAO (mainly A isoform) and COMT (see Table 1.2). The main CNS metabolite of NA is 3-methoxy-4-hydroxy-phenylglycol (MHPG). This is in contrast to the periphery where the main metabolite is vanillylmandelic acid (VMA).

▦ NA release is under inhibitory feedback regulation by terminal α_2-autoreceptors.

Adrenoceptors

▦ The receptors on which NA acts are divided into α- and β-adrenoceptors with further subdivisions within these two main groups. All are G-protein coupled.

▦ Both α_1- and α_2-adrenoreceptors are found within the brain at post-synaptic sites. The α_2 adrenoceptor is also located on noradrenergic terminals and noradrenergic cell bodies where it acts as the autoreceptor.

▦ α_1-Adrenoceptors are excitatory and use inositol phosphate as the second messenger.

▦ α_2-Adrenoceptors are inhibitory and are negatively linked to adenylate cyclase (i.e. they inhibit cAMP production). Clonidine is an α_2-adrenoceptor agonist which is used in the management of morphine withdrawal. It is believed to act presynaptically to reduce withdrawal-related increases in NA release.

▦ β-Adrenoceptors (β_1, β_2, β_3) are stimulatory and positively linked to adenylate cyclase (i.e. they increase cAMP). Antagonists of β-adrenoceptors (β-blockers) have been used in the treatment of anxiety (particularly performance anxiety) based on their central and peripheral actions, leading to reduced autonomic symptoms.

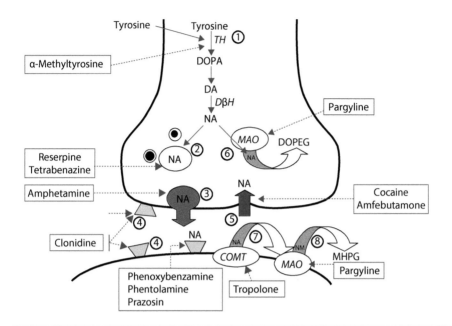

Figure 1.9 Schematic of a central noradrenergic terminal indicating possible sites of drug action. Tyrosine hydroxylase can be blocked by α-methyltyrosine, while DA β-hydroxylase activity is blocked by disulfiram (1). Reserpine and tetrabenazine interfere with the synaptic vesicles, preventing storage of the transmitter. The depletion of NA produced by reserpine is long-lasting and the storage vesicles are irreversibly damaged. Tetrabenazine also interferes with the uptake and/or storage mechanism, but the effects are reversible (2). Amphetamine causes release of NA from the vesicles after entering the terminal via the reuptake transporter NAT (3). Receptors are located on the presynaptic terminal (α_2 autoreceptors) and on the postsynaptic neuron (α_1, α_2, β_1, β_2). Clonidine, an α_2 receptor agonist, reduces NA release by stimulating autoreceptors. Yohimbine and piperoxane are selective α_2 antagonists. Phenoxybenzamine and phenotolamine are α_1-receptor antagonists (4). NA has its action terminated by uptake. The uptake transporter is blocked by tricyclic antidepressants (TCAs) such as desipramine, as well as by reboxetine, venlafaxine and duloxetine and cocaine (5). NA in the cytosol of the terminal is vulnerable to degradation by the enzyme MAO. Pargyline is an effective inhibitor of MAO (6). NA can be inactivated to normetanephrine (NM) by the membrane-bound enzyme catechol-O-methyl transferase (COMT) (7). Tropolone is an inhibitor of COMT. The normetanephrine (NM) formed by the action of COMT on NE can be further metabolised by MAO to MHPG (8).

Serotonin (5-hydroxytryptamine)

Pathways and functions (Figure 1.5)

- The cell bodies of neurons containing 5-HT are located in the mid-brain and brainstem *raphe nuclei*. The dorsal and median raphe nuclei send long ascending projections via the median forebrain bundle. The raphe obscurus, magnus and pallidus send descending projections.
- The *ascending pathways* innervate many forebrain regions including the hippocampus, striatum, amygdala and hypothalamus and cerebral cortex.
  - The terminal fields of dorsal and median raphe projections overlap, but some regions have innervation derived predominantly from the dorsal raphe (e.g. frontal cortex) or median raphe (e.g. dorsal hippocampus).
  - 5-HT has a wide modulatory role in various aspects of behaviour including mood and emotion, sleep/wakefulness and regulation of circadian functions, control of feeding and sexual behaviours, body temperature, cognition, perceptions and emesis.
- The *descending pathways* terminate in the dorsal horn of the spinal cord where they are involved in the inhibition of pain transmission, and the ventral horn where they regulate motor neuron output.

Synthesis and metabolism (Table 1.2, Figure 1.10)

- 5-HT is synthesised from the amino acid tryptophan, by the action of the enzyme tryptophan hydroxylase (TPH), which converts tryptophan to 5-hydroxytryptophan (5-HTP), and 5-HTP decarboxylase, which converts 5-HTP to 5-HT (see Table 1.2).
- TPH is the rate-limiting enzyme in the synthesis of 5-HT and importantly is not saturated by the normal concentrations of tryptophan. Therefore, both increasing and decreasing availability of brain tryptophan will alter brain 5-HT concentration.
- Tryptophan enters the brain in competition with other amino acids, via the large neutral amino acid–facilitated transport system:
  - Administration of a single competing large neutral amino acid such as valine competitively blocks tryptophan transport into the brain.
  - Administration of mixtures of amino acids, lacking in tryptophan, also promotes protein synthesis and so reduces plasma tryptophan which reduces the ratio of tryptophan to competing amino acids.

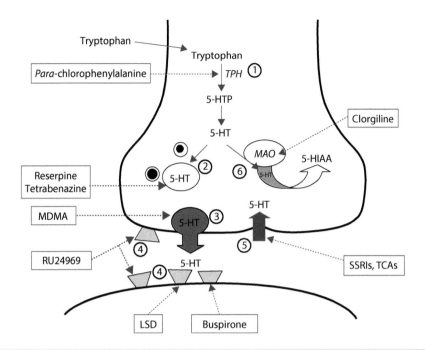

Figure 1.10 Schematic of a central serotonergic terminal indicating possible sites of drug action. Tryptophan is converted to 5-hydroxytryptophan (5-HTP) by tryptophan hydroxylase (1), and this enzyme can be inhibited by *para*-chlorophenylalanine (*p*CPA). 5-HTP is then converted to 5-HT and stored in vesicles (2) protected from degradation by MAO. The vesicles can be disrupted by reserpine and tetrabenazine. *Para*-chloramphetamine, fenfluramine and MDMA can enter 5-HT terminals via the transporter and cause the release of the transmitter from its vesicles (3). 5-HT receptors are located on both pre- and postsynaptic membranes. Presynaptically, 5-HT$_{1B}$ autoreceptors negatively regulate 5-HT release. Postsynpatic receptors include 5-HT$_{1A-F}$, 5-HT$_{2A/C}$ and 5-HT$_3$ subtypes (4). After release, 5-HT is taken up into the terminal by the reuptake transporter (SERT) (5). This is the site of action of many antidepressant drugs including tricyclic antidepressants (TCAs) and selective serotonin reuptake inhibitors (SSRIs). 5-HT in the terminal is metabolised to 5-hydroxyindole acetic acid (5-HIAA) by MAO-A and aldehyde dehydrogenase (6). This process can be blocked by monoamine oxidase inhibitors (MAOIs) including clorgyline and pargyline.

- Thus, it is possible to lower brain 5-HT by reducing plasma tryptophan and/or by *flooding* the transport carrier with other amino acids. These two methods have been exploited in studies in humans to investigate the function of brain 5-HT.

5-HT is stored in vesicles protected from MAO and is released in response to depolarisation of the nerve terminal. 5-HT is mainly metabolised by MAO-A but MAO-B also plays a role and this may be greater when MAO-A is blocked.

▦ The major mechanism for removing 5-HT from the synaptic cleft is re-uptake by the 5-HT transporter (5-HTT). 5-HTT is inhibited by SSRIs and tricyclic antidepressants. There are two well-described polymorphisms of the 5-HTT gene:
  – The variable number tandem repeat (VNTR) is a repeated sequence in the second intron.
  – The serotonin transporter–linked promoter polymorphic region (5-HTTLPR) is a repeat sequence in the promoter region of the gene which influences the activity of the transporter.
  – In addition, single nucleotide polymorphisms (SNPs) also occur. Some studies indicate that these polymorphisms (particularly 5-HTTLPR) may influence vulnerability to depression and/or anti-depressant treatment response.
▦ 5-HT is metabolised intraneuronally by MAO to form 5-hydroxyindole acetic acid (5-HIAA), which is actively transported across the blood–brain barrier, out of the brain.
▦ 5-HT release at the terminals is subject to inhibitory autoregulation involving $5\text{-}HT_{1B}$ and $5\text{-}HT_{1D}$ receptors.

5-HT receptors (Figure 1.11)

▦ There are 14 known 5-HT receptors, all are G-protein coupled except the $5\text{-}HT_3$ subtype which is a ligand-gated cation channel.
▦ $5\text{-}HT_1$ receptors ($5\text{-}HT_{1A}$, $5\text{-}HT_{1B}$, $5\text{-}HT_{1D}$) are inhibitory and are negatively coupled to adenylate cyclase. $5\text{-}HT_{1A}$ receptors also couple to ion channels (G-protein-linked inward rectifying potassium channel [GIRK] and Ca^{2+} channels).
  – $5\text{-}HT_{1A}$ receptors are found both at somatodendritic and postsynaptic sites. Somatodendritic $5\text{-}HT_{1A}$ receptors in the dorsal and median raphe nuclei are autoreceptors regulating 5-HT neuronal firing. Postsynaptic $5\text{-}HT_{1A}$ receptors are found in various brain regions including the hippocampus and PAG where importantly, they regulate behaviours such as resilience, impulsivity and restraint of excessive response to stress as well as aspects of cognitive function. The $5\text{-}HT_{1A}$ receptor may be an important target in the action of antidepressants.
  – $5\text{-}HT_2$ receptors ($5\text{-}HT_{2A}$, $5\text{-}HT_{2B}$, $5\text{-}HT_{2C}$) are excitatory and act through the phospholipase C/inositol phosphate pathway. $5\text{-}HT_{2A}$ receptors are found in the cortex and are associated with sensory perception. The hallucinogen LSD is a $5\text{-}HT_{2A}$ receptor partial agonist. Activation of $5\text{-}HT_{2C}$ receptors can reduce food intake and induce anxiety/panic.
▦ $5\text{-}HT_3$ receptors are excitatory ligand-gated ion channels and are found in high density in the area postrema and nucleus tractus solitarius. $5\text{-}HT_3$ receptor antagonists (e.g. ondansetron) have their anti-emetic actions in this region. $5\text{-}HT_3$ receptors are also known to regulate DA release in the nucleus accumbens.

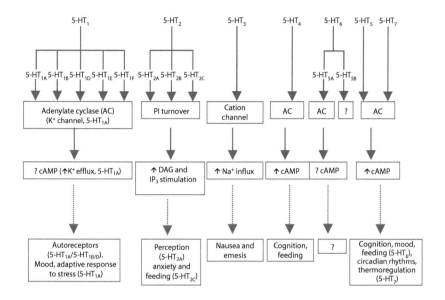

Figure 1.11 Summary of the types of 5-HT receptors, their receptor coupling mechanisms and proposed functions.

- The 5-HT$_4$, 5-HT$_5$, 5-HT$_6$ and 5-HT$_7$ receptors are positively coupled to adenylate cyclase and are thus excitatory. 5-HT$_6$ receptor antagonists have been shown, in animal studies, to modulate memory and attention and are currently in clinical trials for their cognitive effects, while the 5-HT$_7$ receptor may have importance in depression and circadian functions.

Acetylcholine

Pathways and functions (Figure 1.5)

- The distribution of ACh neuronal cell bodies in the brain is more diffuse than that of the catecholamines and 5-HT.
- Cholinergic nuclei are located in the basal forebrain and in the pons. The most important nuclei with regard to psychopharmacology are the *nucleus basalis of Meynert* which projects to the cortex, and the *lateral septum* which sends a projection to the hippocampus (*septohippocampal pathway*). This latter pathway is disrupted in Alzheimer's disease and appears associated with the consequent memory dysfunction.
- Cholinergic nuclei in the midbrain (the *pedunculopontine nucleus* and *laterodorsal tegmental nucleus*) innervate the thalamus and appear to be involved in sleep.
- Many regions including the striatum contain short cholinergic interneurons (see Figure 1.5).

Synthesis and metabolism (Table 1.2, Figure 1.10)

- ACh is synthesised from choline and acetyl coenzyme-A (CoA), a reaction which is catalysed by the enzyme choline acetyltransferase (ChAT) (Table 1.2, Figure 1.12).
- ACh is stored in vesicles in the nerve terminals and is released when the terminal is depolarised.
- Following release ACh is metabolised by acetylcholinesterase (AChE) to form choline and free acetate. Choline is taken up into the nerve

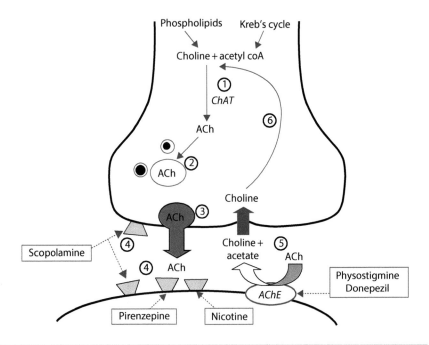

Figure 1.12 Schematic of a central cholinergic terminal indicating possible sites of drug action. ACh is synthesised from choline and acetyl-coA by ChAT. ACh is stored in vesicles, but there are no clinically effective drugs that act at this site (2). There is some evidence that aminopyridines and phosphatidylserines release ACh and may have limited use in Alzheimer's disease patients (3). Presynaptic muscarinic M_2 autoreceptors (4) negatively regulate ACh release. Antagonists at these receptors may have the potential in the treatment of Alzheimer's disease, but existing drugs have poor brain penetration and short half-lives. Postsynaptic receptors are of both muscarinic and nicotinic subtypes. In the synaptic cleft, ACh is broken down by AChE to form acetate and choline. AChE is a major target for the pharmacotherapy of Alzheimer's disease, but to date, AChE inhibitors show only limited efficacy in mild-to-moderate dementia (5). Choline is transported back into the neuron and recycled (6).

terminal by an active transport system and can then be re-used to synthesise ACh.

- Drugs that inhibit AChE are used in the symptomatic treatment of Alzheimer's disease (see Chapter 9).

Cholinergic receptors

- These are subdivided into two classes: Nicotinic and muscarinic, with further subdivision within the classes.
- Nicotinic receptors (nAChRs) are involved in fast excitatory synaptic transmission and are directly coupled to cation channels.
  - They are pentameric structures comprising α and β subunits.
  - There are two basic types: Muscle (found at the neuromuscular junction) and neuronal (widespread in the CNS).
  - In the brain, receptors composed of α_4 and β_2 subunits ($\alpha_4\beta_2$) and receptors composed entirely of α_7 subunits (α_7 homomers) are the most common although $\alpha_3\beta_4$ are also present.
  - The different receptor subtypes have different distributions and distinct pharmacology.
  - Effects of nicotine on CNS nicotinic receptors in the substantia nigra are considered to be responsible for the rewarding (and addictive) properties of smoking.
- There are five muscarinic receptors (M_1–M_5), all found in the brain:
  - They are G-protein coupled and either activate formation of IP_3 (M_1, M_3, M_5) or inhibit cAMP (M_2, M_4).
  - M_1 receptor agonists and M_2 (autoreceptor) antagonists offer potential targets for the treatment of Alzheimer's disease.

γ-Aminobutyric acid

Organisation and functions, synthesis and metabolism (Table 1.2)

- Short GABA neurons (so-called *interneurons*) are widely distributed within the brain with the highest densities in the basal ganglia, hypothalamus, amygdala and other limbic areas. There are also long GABAergic projection neurons in the brain. For example, the projection from the striatum to the substantia nigra which is affected in Huntington's chorea is GABAergic.
- GABA is formed by decarboxylation of glutamate, catalysed by the enzyme glutamic acid decarboxylase (GAD) which exists in two isoforms (GAD65 and GAD67). GABA is taken up into synaptic vesicles by the *vesicular GABA transporter* (VGAT) which also transports glycine (see Section GABA receptors).

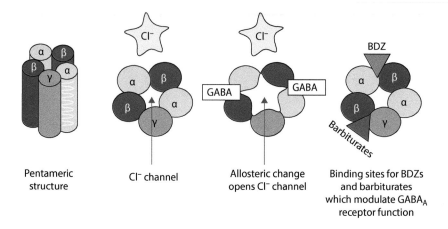

| Pentameric structure | Cl⁻ channel | Allosteric change opens Cl⁻ channel | Binding sites for BDZs and barbiturates which modulate GABA$_A$ receptor function |

Figure 1.13 The GABA$_A$ receptor complex is a pentameric structure composed of α_2, β, and (usually) γ subunits arranged to form a central pore. Activation of the GABA$_A$ receptor by GABA or agonists causes a conformational change, opening the pore and allowing Cl⁻ ions to flow into the cell, causing membrane hyperpolarisation. The GABA$_A$ receptor complex has multiple binding sites. Benzodiazepines are agonists at a site which modulate the ability of GABA to bind to its own site. Agonists at this site facilitate GABA binding, whereas inverse-agonists reduce it. Barbiturates, neurosteroids and ethanol also modulate GABA$_A$ receptor function. Bicuculline is an antagonist of the GABA$_A$-binding site, while muscimol is an agonist at that site. There are multiple forms of each subunit, and receptors composed of the different subunits have different brain distributions and functions. For example, receptors containing α_1-subunits mediate sedation, whilst those containing α_3 subunits mediate anxiolysis. Drugs which can distinguish between receptors with the various subunit isoforms hold promise as selective non-sedating anxiolytics and anticonvulsants.

▦   Following release, GABA can either be taken up into the nerve terminals by a specific transport system or it enters glial cells where it undergoes mitochondrial metabolism, back to glutamate (*GABA shunt*) (see Table 1.2).

▦   The major psychopharmacological interest in GABA is the role of the GABA$_A$ receptor complex in the action of benzodiazepines (BDZ), barbiturates, alcohol and neurosteroids (Figure 1.13 and see Chapter 6).

GABA receptors

▦   GABA acts on two types of receptor: The GABA$_A$ receptor which is a ligand-gated ion channel, and the G-protein-linked GABA$_B$ receptor.

▦   GABA$_A$ receptors are composed of five subunits, each of which can occur in multiple isoforms. Usually, there are two α, two β and a single γ subunit. There are six known α subunit isoforms, three β isoforms and two γ subunit isoforms. Receptors of different subunit composition have different pharmacologies (Figure 1.13).

- The $GABA_A$ receptor (or more correctly '$GABA_A$ receptor complex') is directly coupled to a Cl^- ion channel, and its activation results in an influx of Cl^- and rapid hyperpolarisation (causing neuronal inhibition).
- Barbiturates bind to a site on the $GABA_A$ receptor complex and increase the probability of channel opening in response to GABA, resulting in increased neuronal inhibition. At high concentrations, they can have direct actions in the absence of GABA and hence cause respiratory depression in overdose.
- BDZs bind to a separate site on the $GABA_A$ receptor complex and facilitate the action of GABA, so increasing the frequency of Cl^- channel opening. Because they require GABA to be present for their action, BDZs are less toxic in overdose than barbiturates.
  - BDZs are agonists at their binding sites and their actions can be blocked by antagonists (e.g. flumazenil), while inverse-agonists at the BDZ site decrease GABA transmission (see Figure 1.13)
  - Newer hypnotics such as zopiclone have similar actions to BDZs but interact with specific subtypes of the $GABA_A$ receptor which may reduce the adverse effects (such as memory loss, dependence)
- The $GABA_A$ receptor complex is also modulated by ethanol and neurosteroids which acts at distinct sites.
- $GABA_B$ receptors are found in the brain at both presynaptic and postsynaptic sites. These receptors produce slow inhibitory potentials through an increase in K^+ conductance (GIRK) and inhibit adenylate cyclase. The physiological and behavioural significance of these receptors is not well understood, but they may be important in the absence of seizures, cognitive performance and the regulation of amine release.

Glutamate

Organisation and functions, synthesis and metabolism (Table 1.2)

- Glutamate (an *'excitatory amino acid'*) is the major fast-acting excitatory neurotransmitter in the brain.
- The ubiquitous presence of glutamate in neurons and glial cells in the brain (see below) has hampered the identification of glutamatergic neurons and pathways. However, it is now established that the cell bodies of glutamatergic neurons are widely distributed in the brain. The pyramidal cells of the cerebral cortex and of the hippocampus are glutamatergic.
- Glutamatergic pyramidal neurons in the cerebral cortex project to other cortical regions and to subcortical areas. The perforant path from the entorhinal cortex to the hippocampus is also glutamatergic.

Monoaminergic nuclei in the midbrain and pons are innervated by glutamatergic pathways from the cerebral cortex.

▨ Glutamate is synthesised from glucose in the Kreb's cycle. This metabolic pathway is present in all cells: Glutamate is present in all neurons and glial cells of the CNS. Glutamate can also be synthesised from glutamine: A reaction catalysed by glutaminase, a mitochondrial enzyme expressed in glutamatergic neuron terminals. Although glutamate synthesis takes place in all neurons and glia, glutamatergic neurons uniquely express the *vesicular glutamate transporters* VGLUT1 and VGLUT2 which sequester glutamate into synaptic vesicles. A third type of vesicular glutamate transporter, VGLUT3, is found in non-glutamatergic neurons.

▨ The action of glutamate in the synapse is terminated by one of the high-affinity plasma membrane *excitatory amino acid transporters* (EAAT1–4), also known as glutamate transporters (GluT) which have distinct distributions in both glutamatergic neurons and glia in the brain.

▨ Glutamate taken up into glial cells (via EAAT1 or 2) is metabolised to glutamine which is released and taken up into neighbouring glutamatergic terminals via the low-affinity system A transporter. Thus, glial cells play an important role in the recycling of glutamate.

▨ Glutamate taken up into neurons (via EAAT3 or 4) may be recycled for release.

▨ Two major basic science reasons for the growing interest in brain glutamate are
   – The link between glutamate (NMDA) receptor activation and long-term potentiation (LTP) in the hippocampus as the physiological substrate of memory
   – The link between excessive glutamate receptor activation and neurodegeneration caused by loss of intracellular Ca^{2+} homeostasis

▨ Clinically, there is interest in the role of glutamate transmission in psychosis (schizophrenia), anxiety and depression. The dissociative anaesthetic agents, ketamine and the psychotomimetic phencyclidine (PCP or 'angel dust'), are antagonists at NMDA receptors. Ketamine has been shown to have rapid-onset anti-suicidal and antidepressant properties (see Chapter 4).

Glutamate receptors

▨ Glutamate acts on both ligand-gated ion channels (NMDA, amino-3-hydroxy-5-methyl-4-isoxazole propionate [AMPA] and kainate receptors), and on G-protein-linked metabotropic receptors (mGluR1–8).

▨ AMPA, NMDA and kainate receptors comprise four protein subunits. AMPA consists of GluA1–4 subunits, kainate of GluK1–5 subunits, whilst the NMDA receptor is made of GluN1, GluN2A-D and GluN3A-B subunits.

Note: The nomenclature of glutamate receptor subunits was standardised by IUPHAR in 2010 (see References).

▦ AMPA receptors are permeable to Na^+, whilst NMDA receptors are permeable to both Na^+ and Ca^{2+}. The latter receptor is blocked by magnesium (Mg^{2+}) ions and has an allosteric site that binds glycine.

▦ Metabotropic glutamate receptors are divided into three groups: Group I (mGluR1 and mGluR5), group II (mGluR2 andmGluR3) and group III (mGluR4, mGluR6, mGluR7 and mGluR8). Drugs acting at mGluRs can influence excitotoxicity and epileptiform activity.

Glycine

Organisation and functions, synthesis and metabolism

▦ Glycine is an inhibitory amino acid neurotransmitter in the central and peripheral nervous systems.

▦ The highest densities of glycinergic neuronal cell bodies are found in the spinal cord, brain stem, medulla and retina. They are also found in other regions including the auditory midbrain, hypothalamus and tectum.

▦ Glycinergic axon terminals are widespread in the brain. In the forebrain, the highest densities are found in hippocampus, thalamic nuclei and septum.

▦ In CNS neurons, glycine is thought to be mainly synthesised from serine. This folate-dependent, reversible, reaction is catalysed by serine hydroxymethyltransferase.

▦ Following its synthesis within glycinergic terminals, glycine is sequestered into synaptic vesicles by the action of the *vesicular inhibitory amino acid transporter* (VIAAT) (the same as/also known as VGAT). In some neurons, glycine and GABA may act as co-transmitters and can be stored in, and released from, the same vesicles.

▦ The action of glycine in the synaptic cleft is terminated by two high-affinity plasma membrane *glycine transporters* (GlyT1 and GlyT2): The former is found in glial cells, and the latter in glycinergic neuronal terminals.

▦ Glycine taken up into neurons can then be re-packaged into synaptic vesicles. In glia, glycine is converted to serine.

Glycine receptors

▦ Glycine receptors are tetrameric ligand-gated ion channel receptors composed of α and β subunits. Different hetero- and homomeric variants exist and may confer different pharmacological properties.

- Ligand-activated receptors are permeable to chloride (Cl-) ions which flow into the cell, causing hyperpolarisation of the plasma membrane.
- Glycine receptor activity is modulated by neurosteroids as well as by zinc (Zn^{2+}) ions.
- Glycine and taurine are both agonists for glycine receptors. The alkaloid strychnine is an antagonist of glycine receptors and causes pychostimulation and violent clonic seizures by blocking glycinergic inhibitory tone centrally and within the ventral horn of the spinal cord.
- In the CNS (but not in the spinal cord), glycine also acts as a co-agonist along with glutamate at the NMDA receptor where it promotes excitatory neurotransmission. There is interest in glycinergic drugs for the treatment of schizophrenia, including negative symptoms.

Bibliography

Bear MF, Connors BW, Paradiso MA. *Neuroscience Exploring the Brain*, 3rd edn. Baltimore, MD: Lippincott, Williams & Wilkins, 2006.

Hammond C. *Cellular and Molecular Neurobiology*, 23rd edn. London, UK: Academic Press, 2008.

International Union of Basic and Clinical Pharmacology (IUPHAR). Revised recommendations for nomenclature of ligand-gated ion channels, 2010. http://www.guidetopharmacology.org/LGICNomenclature.jsp.

Iversen LL, Iversen SD, Bloom FE, Roth RH. *Introduction to Neuropsychopharmacology*. Oxford, UK: OUP, 2009.

Leonard BE. *Fundamentals of Psychopharmacology*, 3rd edn. Chichester, UK: John Wiley, 2003.

Rang HP, Dale MM, Ritter R, Flower G, Henderson PK. *Pharmacology*, 7th edn. Edinburgh, UK: Churchill Livingstone, 2011.

Shiloh R, Stryjer R, Nutt D, Weizman A. *Atlas of Psychiatric Pharmacotherapy*, 2nd edn. London, UK: Taylor & Francis Group, 2006.

Pharmacokinetics and pharmacodynamics

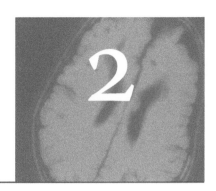

Ian M Anderson

 ## Pharmacokinetics

Basics

- Pharmacokinetics is concerned with the time course and disposition of drugs in the body ('the body's effect on drugs').
- Drugs are intended to act on target organs but usually have to be given systemically.
- Targeted organ delivery methods include tissue-specific 'activation' (e.g. metabolism of the prodrug levodopa to DA in neurons) and implanted drug-coated devices.
- Movement of drug molecules into and around the body occurs by
  - *Bulk flow* (in blood, lymph and cerebrospinal fluid) which is independent of drug chemistry
  - Traversing barriers by *diffusion* and *active transport* which depend on drug chemistry
- Important barriers formed by layers of cells include those between the body and the environment (*epithelium*) and between blood and organs (vascular *endothelium*).
  - Drug movement can be through gaps between cells (not present in the epithelium nor the capillaries of the *blood–brain barrier* [BBB]) or across *cell membranes.*
  - Cell membranes consist of *lipoproteins*, allowing lipid-soluble molecules to diffuse across them down a *concentration gradient.*
  - Non-lipid-soluble molecules cross cell membranes through *carrier mechanisms* (most important for drugs) or *aqueous channels* (limited to very small molecules such as gases).

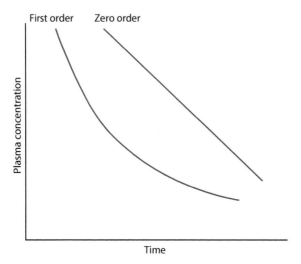

Figure 2.1   In elimination with zero-order kinetics, concentration falls steadily in a straight line, whereas with first-order kinetics, the curve is exponential.

- *Bioavailability* (how much of an administered drug reaches its target) is determined by three main factors:
  - Absorption
  - Distribution
  - Elimination (metabolism and/or excretion)
- *First-order kinetics* (Figure 2.1) results from the *law of mass action* which states that 'the rate of a reaction is proportional to the active masses of the reacting substances'. The rate of absorption or elimination is directly proportional to the amount of drug remaining. This applies to most psychotropic drugs.
- With *zero-order kinetics* (Figure 2.1), a fixed amount of drug is absorbed or eliminated for each unit of time independent of drug concentrations, because of some other rate-limiting factor. Also known as *nonlinear kinetics* clinically. Examples are the metabolism of alcohol and phenytoin (saturation of metabolic enzymes) and absorption of controlled release drugs and depot antipsychotics. Drug elimination can change from first- to zero-order at high enough doses if the metabolic pathway becomes saturated (e.g. some tricyclic antidepressants [TCAs]).
- Following drug administration, there is a rise and fall in plasma concentration determined by the processes of absorption, distribution and elimination (see Figure 2.2).
  - C_{max} is the maximum plasma concentration achieved.

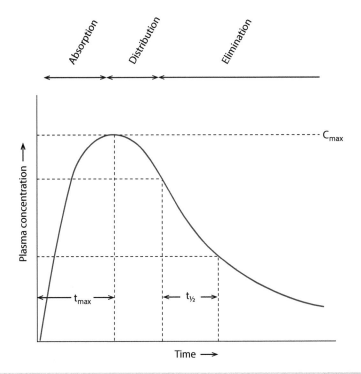

Figure 2.2 Plasma drug concentration in the phases of absorption, distribution and elimination.

- t_{max} is the time at which C_{max} occurs after administration (tends to be variable between individuals).
- $t_{½}$ is the time for the plasma concentration to fall by a half (elimination half-life).
- The area under the curve (AUC) after a single dose is proportional to the amount of drug in plasma and allows determination of fraction of dose absorbed – the bioavailability.

Different routes of drug administration and relevant features are described in Table 2.1.

Absorption

- Absorption is influenced by the route of administration and drug properties.
- C_{max} is inversely proportional to t_{max} for a given AUC.
- Drug delivery systems that control drug release to modify absorption (i.e. increase t_{max}) allow the reduction of peak blood concentrations (C_{max})

Table 2.1   Comparison of routes of drug administration

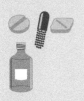
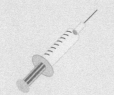
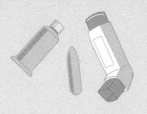

Oral	Parenteral	Others
Most common route but leads to variable plasma concentration because Absorption may be erratic. Drugs are subject to metabolism by liver (*first-pass effect*). To be absorbed, drugs must be Soluble in gastro-intestinal fluids Acid resistant Able to pass across cell membranes which occurs by passive diffusion and is dependent on lipid solubility Gastric juice is strongly acid, causing weak acids to be unionised and readily absorbed (vice versa for weak alkalis)	*Intravenous* Most rapid method *Intramuscular* Absorption occurs over 10–30 min. Rate is dependent on Blood flow. Aqueous solubility. Long-acting injectable preparations with slow absorption; examples include solutions of drugs in inert oil ('depot'), encapsulated microspheres and pamoate salts. *Others* Include subcutaneous, intrathecal, etc., not currently used in psychiatric practice	Infrequently used in psychiatric practice. Includes: Transcutaneous Across mucous membranes, e.g. sublingual, rectal Inhalation

and more prolonged action (e.g. delayed release tablets, intramuscular depot preparations).

▪ Liquid preparations (e.g. risperidone and fluoxetine) and oral dispersible tablets (e.g. olanzapine, risperidone and mirtazapine) are aimed at ensuring administration/improving compliance. They generally have minimal effects on absorption.

▪ Absorption that bypasses the gut and liver avoids *first-pass metabolism* by the liver, allowing a greater proportion of the dose to be available systemically, and reducing any gut-mediated effects (e.g. transdermal selegiline).

Distribution (Figure 2.3)

- During the (re)distribution phase in plasma, the drug is distributed to various tissues in the body depending on
  - Plasma protein binding
  - Tissue perfusion
  - Permeability of tissue membranes
  - Active transport out of tissues (P-glycoprotein)
- Distribution leads to a fall in plasma concentration and is most rapid after intravenous administration.
- Distribution can be viewed as the drug achieving equilibrium between different compartments. An approximation is the two-compartment model: Central compartment (plasma) and peripheral compartment (tissues).
- The apparent *volume of distribution* ($V_d = Q/C_p$) tells us about the characteristics of a drug (V_d = volume of distribution; Q = quantity of drug; C_p = plasma concentration). When V_d is high, it indicates that the drug has high affinity for tissues outside body water such as brain and fat.
- Drugs may be bound to sites where they exert no effect but which influence distribution and elimination:
  - Plasma proteins – If highly bound to these, drugs (e.g. many antidepressants, anticonvulsants and warfarin) may displace each other, leading to increased free plasma concentration
  - Fat and other sites that may only release drugs slowly, leading to persistence of drugs in the body (e.g. antipsychotics)

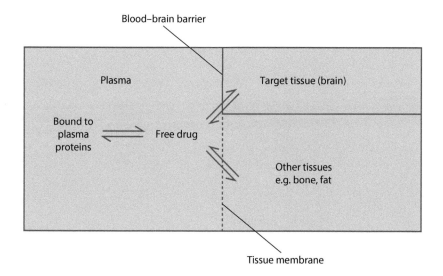

Figure 2.3 Distribution of drug between different body 'compartments'.

- *BBB*, as a consequence of tight junctions between the capillary endo-
  thelial cells, only allows lipid-soluble molecules into the brain (most
  psychotropic drugs are lipid soluble).
    - Non-lipid-soluble drugs require special transport systems that can
      be active (e.g. L-tryptophan, L-dopa) or passive (e.g. lithium).
    - *P-glycoprotein* is an endothelial membrane protein which pumps drugs
      out of capillary cells by an ATP-dependent process and effectively pre-
      vents some drugs getting into the brain (e.g. the opioid loperamide).
    - Areas of brain not protected by the BBB include the median emi-
      nence of the hypothalamus and the vomiting centre.
    - Inflammation makes the BBB more permeable to molecules that
      are otherwise prevented from entering the brain.

Elimination (Figure 2.4)

Metabolism

- Metabolism by the liver is most important, but it may also occur in
  plasma, lung and kidney.
- In general, metabolism converts lipid-soluble psychotropic drugs to
  water-soluble compounds to facilitate elimination.
- Metabolism is usually the rate-limiting step that determines the kinetics of a drug (an exception is lithium that is eliminated unaltered).
- Metabolism is often divided into two phases:
    - *Phase I* (or non-synthetic) metabolism involves modification of a drug
      which may make it more or less active than the parent compound.

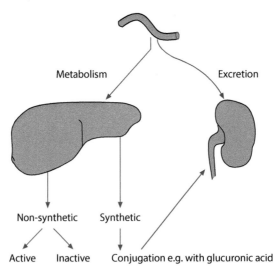

Figure 2.4 Main routes of elimination of a drug.

- *Phase II* (or synthetic) metabolism involves conjugation of a drug with another large molecule to make it water soluble and inactive.
- Phase I metabolism:
  - This consists of oxidation, reduction, hydrolysis and demethylation by two main enzyme systems, *cytochrome P450* (CYP450, or CYP) and *flavin-containing mono-oxygenase* (FMO).
  - The CYP family of hepatic enzymes is responsible for the oxidative metabolism of most psychotropic drugs; the dominant isoenzyme in drug metabolism is CYP3A4 (see Table 2.2 for the most important isoenzymes and examples of their metabolites).
  - There is a genetic variation in hepatic enzymes, affecting the rate of metabolism. The most studied is CYP2D6. About 5%–10% of Caucasians, but only 1%–2% of Asians, lack this enzyme and are *poor metabolisers* of the probe drug substrate, dextromethorphan. There are also *extensive metabolisers* of dextromethorphan. In contrast, up to 25% of East Asians are poor metabolisers for CYP2C19. The genotyping for some CYP isoenzymes (*pharmacogenetics*) is now clinically available, but its utility is still unclear.
  - *N*-oxygenation by FMO which is grouped into five families (1–5). FMO appears less important in drug metabolism than CYP, is rarely inhibited by compounds, and is implicated less in toxic reactions. Substrates include clozapine and olanzapine.
- Phase II metabolism is usually conjugation with glucuronic acid by uridine diphosphate glucuronosyltransferases (UDPGT), of which families 1 and 2 are most important for the glucuronidation of drugs. Conjugation can also occur with other charged compounds such as glutathione and glycine.
- Factors influencing metabolism:
  - Genetic variation in the activity of CYP enzymes (see the previous text).
  - The number of enzyme pathways involved (e.g. sertraline is metabolised by multiple pathways, reducing the influence of individual CYP enzymes).
  - Drug–drug interactions, leading to inhibition or induction of CYP enzymes (resulting in decreased and increased metabolism, respectively) (see Table 2.2). Examples include fluoxetine increasing plasma TCA concentrations, fluvoxamine increasing plasma clozapine concentrations, carbamazepine decreasing plasma concentration of many drugs (including contraceptive pill).
  - Drug interactions leading to inhibition or induction of glucuronidation: For example valproate reduces lamotrigine glucuronidation, leading to increased plasma concentrations.
  - Drugs competing for same metabolic pathway (decreasing metabolism of both).
  - Impaired liver function due to increased age and liver impairment (decreases metabolism).

Table 2.2 Main cytochrome P450 (CYP450) isoenzymes with examples of important psychotropic drug substrates, inducers and inhibitors

	CYP450 isoenzymes				
	1A2	2C9	2C19	2D6	3A3/4
Substrates	Clozapine Duloxetine Haloperidol Olanzapine TCAs	Phenytoin Warfarin Fluoxetine	Citalopram Diazepam TCAs	Aripiprazole Citalopram Donepezil Duloxetine Galantamine Fluoxetine Paroxetine Risperidone TCAs Typical antipsychotics Venlafaxine Vortioxetine	Aripiprazole Benzodiazepines Ca^{2+} channel blockers Carbamazepine Clozapine TCAs Reboxetine Quetiapine
Inducers		Phenobarbitone	Carbamazepine		Carbamazepine Phenytoin
Inhibitors	Fluvoxamine		Fluvoxamine Fluoxetine	Antipsychotics Duloxetine Fluoxetine Paroxetine	Fluoxetine Nefazodone

NB: This list is not comprehensive and it is important to consult a formulary such as the British National Formulary for interactions when prescribing.

Excretion

- Excretion by the kidneys is most important but may also occur through lungs or in bile, sweat, milk and saliva.
- May be of the original drug or its metabolites.
    - Ionised and non-lipid-soluble compounds are excreted best.
    - Lithium is the most important drug to be excreted by the kidneys in an unaltered form.
- Factors influencing excretion:
    - Reduction in renal blood flow (e.g. non-steroidal anti-inflammatory drugs, dehydration) (decreased glomerular filtration)
    - Alteration in reabsorption (urine pH, e.g. alkaline diuresis reduces aspirin reabsorption and increases excretion; low Na^+ increases lithium reabsorption and decreases excretion)
    - Decreased renal function due to renal impairment, increased age

Plasma drug concentrations

- *Steady-state concentration* is achieved after repeated doses lead to an equilibrium between absorption and elimination (Figure 2.5):
    - This is directly dependent on dose and elimination half-life for drugs with first-order kinetics, and it is achieved after 4–5 half-lives.

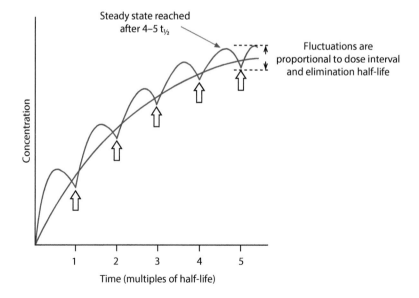

Figure 2.5   Plasma concentration of a drug after repeated administration.

- – Doses given at greater intervals than the half-life lead to large fluctuations in plasma concentration.
- – Drugs with zero-order kinetics show disproportionately large increases in plasma concentration as doses are increased (non-linear kinetics), and may not reach steady-state concentration if absorption is greater than the fixed rate of elimination (e.g. phenytoin).
- – Delayed release preparations, which slow absorption, reduce plasma fluctuations and allow greater intervals between administrations (but do not alter the time to steady-state concentration). This allows once-daily dosing in short-half-life oral drugs (e.g. venlafaxine, quetiapine and lithium), and weekly or longer parenteral administration (e.g. depot antipsychotics).
- Large initial doses (*loading doses*) may be given to achieve therapeutic plasma concentrations more rapidly (e.g. valproate for mania).
- Some drugs have a recognised *therapeutic range* of plasma concentrations (e.g. lithium, many anticonvulsant drugs).
- The *therapeutic index* is the ratio of the minimum plasma drug concentration causing toxic effects to that causing a therapeutic effect. A low therapeutic index (e.g. lithium, phenytoin) usually requires monitoring of plasma/serum concentrations.

Pharmacodynamics

Basics

- Pharmacodynamics is the study of the mechanism of drug action ('the effect of drugs on the body').
- Most psychoactive drugs affect the function of specific neurotransmitters either directly or indirectly (see next section).
- Drugs affecting monoamine neurotransmitters (DA, NA, 5-HT) are important in the treatment of psychotic and affective disorders.
- Drugs acting on amino acid neurotransmitters (GABA and glutamate) have traditionally been important in the treatment of anxiety disorders and epilepsy, and are now being explored for psychotic and affective disorders.
- Drugs enhancing cholinergic function are used to treat dementia.
- There is interest in drugs acting on other neurotransmitters (e.g. peptides, nitric oxide, opioids, cannabinoids).
- Alteration of neurotransmitter function is also commonly responsible for *side effects* (unwanted or adverse effects).
- Drugs may also act at other sites:
  - – *Membrane effects* directly altering neuronal function (e.g. anaesthetics, alcohol)
  - – *Ligand-activated transcription factors* altering gene expression by action on nuclear receptors (e.g. corticosteroids, triiodothyronine)

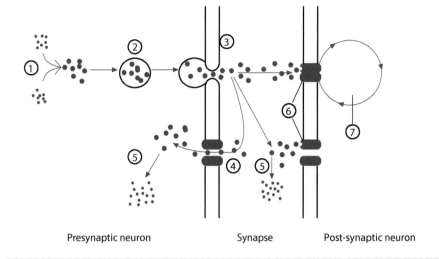

Presynaptic neuron   Synapse   Post-synaptic neuron

Figure 2.6 Sites of drug action on neurotransmitters (for key to numbers see text).

Sites of drug action on neurotransmitters (Figure 2.6)

1. *Synthesis* (e.g. L-tryptophan is the precursor of 5-HT and administration results in increased 5-HT synthesis).
2. *Storage* (e.g. reserpine depletes NA and DA stores in nerve terminal vesicles).
3. *Release* (e.g. amphetamine releases NA and DA into the synapse).
4. *Reuptake* (e.g. TCAs inhibit monoamine reuptake into the presynaptic neuron and so increase neurotransmitter concentration in the synapse).
5. *Degradation* (e.g. monoamine oxidase inhibitors [MAOIs] prevent the breakdown of monoamine neurotransmitters).
6. *Receptors* (e.g. antipsychotics antagonise DA receptors).
7. *Other post-synaptic mechanisms* (e.g. lithium inhibits second messenger function, antagonists of Ca^{2+} channels).

Drug-receptor dynamics

- The *affinity* of a drug for a receptor reflects how strongly it tends to bind to the receptor.
- The *efficacy* of a drug reflects how strongly it tends to activate the receptor after binding.

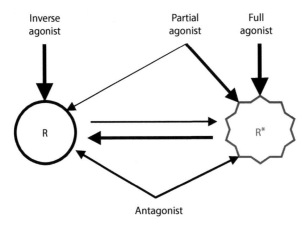

Figure 2.7   Two-state receptor model. When no ligand is present, more receptors are in the 'resting' (R) than the activated (R*) state. Antagonists bind to both R and R*, maintaining the equilibrium and preventing the binding of agonists. Different types of agonists change the balance between R* (full agonists) and R (inverse agonists).

- The *two-state receptor model* proposes that receptors can be in an activated or *resting* state existing in equilibrium, and it is this balance that determines the overall effect of a group of receptors on a neuron (Figure 2.7). However, it is now recognised that receptors may have multiple conformational states with different binding properties and functional effects.
- Receptors may have multiple binding sites (*allosteric sites*) which can influence the action of drugs binding elsewhere on the receptor (e.g. glycine is an allosteric facilitator at the glutamate receptor, benzodiazepines [BDZ] allosterically modify binding of GABA at GABA$_A$ receptors).

Agonists

- *Agonists* are drugs which mimic endogenous neurotransmitters, and bind to the activated form of the receptor, changing the overall receptor equilibrium to favour activation (Figure 2.7).
- Most drugs bind reversibly to receptors, and in the simplest case, the response is proportional to the fraction of receptors occupied (*law of mass action*).
- As the concentration of drug increases, the response increases until all the receptors are occupied, giving a *dose–response curve* as shown in Figure 2.8. When maximum response is achieved without full receptor occupancy, there are said to be *spare receptors*.

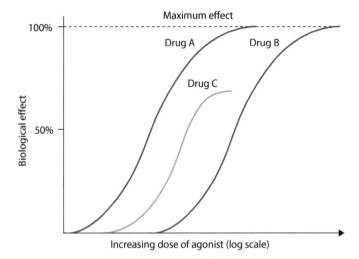

Figure 2.8 Different patterns of responses to agonists (see text for explanation).

- In Figure 2.8, the two *full agonists* (A and B) are able to bring about maximum responses; however, A does so at a lower concentration than B, because it has a greater *affinity* for the receptor.
- Drug C, in Figure 2.8, has a lower *efficacy* than A and B and does not cause a maximal response even when all receptors are occupied, and is a *partial agonist* (e.g. buspirone, buprenorphine, aripiprazole). This can be explained by the two-state receptor model (see Figure 2.7).
- *Inverse agonists* bring about the opposite effects to those seen with agonists (e.g. inverse BDZ agonists decrease, rather than increase, binding of GABA to GABA$_A$ receptors and hence increase anxiety). This occurs when the 'resting' state has intrinsic activity in the opposite direction to the activated state, and preferentially binds the inverse agonist (see Figure 2.7).
- The *potency* of a drug is the amount required to achieve a defined biological effect. It is determined by
  - The proportion of the drug reaching the receptor
  - Its affinity for the receptor
  - Its efficacy at the receptor

Antagonists

- *Antagonists* block the action of agonists (and inverse agonists), causing a reduced effect for a given concentration of agonist or inverse agonist (e.g. a shift to the right in the dose–response curve for an agonist). According to the two-state receptor model, they bind to

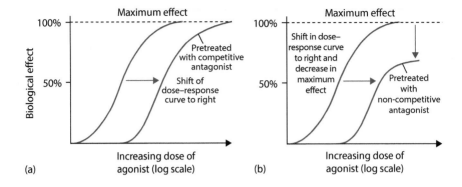

Figure 2.9 Effect of antagonists on the action of agonist drugs (see text for explanation): (a) competitive antagonist, and (b) non-competitive antagonist.

both 'resting' and activated states of receptors without changing the intrinsic equilibrium between the two states, thereby appearing to be neutral in effect. Fully neutral antagonists (i.e. without any agonist or inverse agonist effects) are sometimes called *silent antagonists* (they have affinity for the receptor but no efficacy).

▪ Most antagonist drugs are *competitive* and are displaced from their binding site by agonists so that at high doses the agonist can still exert maximum effect (Figure 2.9a). This competition is influenced by the relative affinity of the agonist and antagonist for the receptor.

▪ *Non-competitive antagonists* cannot be displaced by agonists and not only shift the curve to the right but also reduce the maximum effect (Figure 2.9b). Non-competitive antagonists are called *reversible* if the system is restored to normal when the antagonist is removed (e.g. cyclothiazide binding to an allosteric site on glutamate mGluR1 receptors), and *irreversible* if restoration of function requires synthesis of new receptors/enzymes (e.g. phenelzine binding to monoamine oxidase).

▪ Some antagonists (termed *uncompetitive*) require receptor activation before binding to an allosteric receptor site, so a given amount shows a greater effect at higher, compared to lower, agonist concentrations (e.g. memantine at glutamate NMDA receptors).

▪ In the presence of a full agonist, increasing concentrations of a partial agonist will antagonise the response until the level of its own maximal response is reached (Figure 2.10). Higher doses of a high-affinity, partial agonist therefore 'set' a level of neurotransmission which is independent of the concentration of an agonist. For example it is proposed that aripiprazole 'stabilises' DA neurotransmission (avoiding both over- and underactivity), resulting in benefit to both positive and negative symptoms of schizophrenia, with less propensity to cause EPSE.

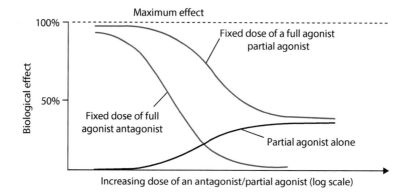

Figure 2.10 Effect of increasing doses of a partial agonist alone and in the presence of a full agonist (see text for explanation).

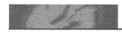

The term *functional antagonist* is sometimes used to describe a drug that indirectly inhibits the effect of receptor activation, rather than through an effect at the receptor itself.

Tolerance and sensitisation

Tolerance describes the diminished response to the administration of a drug after repeated exposure. It may be caused by
- Increased metabolism (e.g. carbamazepine increases the activity of enzymes that metabolise it, i.e. *enzyme induction*)
- Reduced receptor sensitivity or number (*down-regulation*)
- Activation of a *homeostatic* mechanism (e.g. in the second messenger or effector system)
- *Behavioural tolerance* through learning to cope with the effects

Cross-tolerance occurs when tolerance to one drug transfers to another, and can be due to pharmacodynamic (e.g. alcohol and barbiturates) or pharmacokinetic (e.g. carbamazepine and oral contraceptives) reasons.

Sensitisation is the enhancement of drug effects following the repeated administration of the same dose of drug (e.g. as seen in animals after stimulants such as amphetamines).

Bibliography

Cooper JR, Bloom FE, Roth RH. *The Biochemical Basis of Neuropharmacology*, 8th edn. New York: Oxford University Press, 2002.

Rang HP, Dale MM, Ritter JM, Flower RJ, Henderson G. *Rang and Dale's Pharmacology*, 7th edn. Edinburgh, UK: Elsevier Churchill Livingstone, 2012.

Schatzberg AF, Nemeroff CB. *The American Psychiatric Publishing Textbook of Psychopharmacology*, 4th edn. Arlington, TX: American Psychiatric Publishing, Inc., 2009.

Schatzberg AF, Nemeroff CB. *Essentials of Clinical Psychopharmacology*, 3rd edn. Arlington, TX: American Psychiatric Publishing, Inc., 2013.

Shiloh R, Stryjer R, Nutt D, Weizman A. *Atlas of Psychiatric Pharmacotherapy*, 2nd edn. New York: Taylor & Francis Group, 2006.

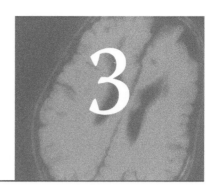

Antipsychotics

Frances Cheng, Peter B Jones and Peter S Talbot

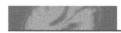
History

Like the antidepressants, antipsychotic drugs were discovered by chance.

- *1950s*: Phenothiazines developed. Chlorpromazine was synthesised originally as an antihistamine/antihelminthic but was found subsequently to be sedative and antipsychotic. More compounds were synthesised within the same and related classes (e.g. thioxanthines; Table 3.1). The butyrophenones were created in the late 1950s: Haloperidol began life as a candidate analgesic, and was later found to have antipsychotic properties. Further compounds were synthesised in this and other classes, for example phenylbutylpiperidine.
- *1960s*: Clozapine synthesised in 1961; currently the most efficacious and prototypical atypical antipsychotic on the basis of few extrapyramidal motor effects in rats.
- *1970s*: Clozapine introduced then was withdrawn in 1975 due to fatal agranulocytosis. Further atypical or second-generation drugs developed (Table 3.2).
- *1980s*: Clozapine 'rediscovered' with recognition of efficacy where other antipsychotics have failed.
- *1990s*: New, second-generation antipsychotics introduced: Amisulpride, olanzapine, quetiapine, risperidone, sertindole, ziprasidone.
- *2000s*: First D_2 receptor partial agonist antipsychotic introduced: Aripiprazole.

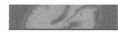
Dopamine hypothesis

The DA system (see Chapter 1) is believed to play an important role in the action of antipsychotic drugs:

- All our currently available first- or second-line drugs share the property of antagonism at the D_2 receptor, and their antipsychotic efficacy is

Table 3.1 Chemical classification of older 'typical' or first-generation antipsychotic drugs

Phenothiazine	
Aliphatic side chain	Chlorpromazine
	Levomepromazine
	Promazine
Piperidine	Thioridazine (withdrawn due to ↑QTc)
	Pipotiazine (depot only, withdrawn due to unavailable ingredient)
Piperazine	Fluphenazine
	Perphenazine
	Prochlorperazine
	Trifluoperazine
Thioxanthene	Flupentixol
	Zuclopenthixol
Butyrophenone	Droperidol (withdrawn due to ↑QTc)
	Haloperidol
Diphenylbutylpiperidine	Pimozide
Substituted benzamide	Sulpiride (NB; clinically relatively atypical, despite its receptor pharmacology)

Table 3.2 Chemical classification of 'atypical' or second-generation antipsychotic drugs

Dibenzodiazepine	Clozapine
Thienobenzodiazepine	Olanzapine
Dibenzothiazepine	Quetiapine
Benzisoxazole	Risperidone, paliperidone, iloperidone
Imidazolidinone	Sertindole
Substituted benzamide	Amisulpride
Quinolinones	Aripiprazole
Benzothiazolylpiperazine	Ziprasidone
Dibenzothiazepine	Zotepine[a]
Dibenzo-oxypino pyrrole	Asenapine
Benzisothiazol	Lurasidone

[a] NB: Zotepine withdrawn from the United Kingdom in 2011.

believed to be due to D_2 receptor antagonism in the striatum (caudate nucleus and putamen).

▨ The classical DA theory hypothesised that psychosis was due to increased DA in the mesolimbic system. This was later extended to include the proposal that cognitive impairment in schizophrenia is associated with decreased DA in dorsolateral prefrontal cortex.

▨ The current version of the hypothesis proposes that psychosis is associated with increased DA presynaptic function in the nigrostriatal pathway (particularly the part that projects to the *associative* subdivision of the striatum) rather than the mesolimbic system. DA abnormalities are believed to be secondary or 'knock-on' effects of a more primary abnormality, perhaps in the glutamate or GABA systems.

Key findings

▨ *1960s*: Antipsychotics found to increase turnover of brain DA.

▨ *1970s*: The greater the DA receptor binding affinity of an antipsychotic, the greater is the clinical potency (Figure 3.1).

▨ *1980s*: α-Flupentixol but not β-flupentixol has antipsychotic activity greater than placebo (only the α-isomer is an antagonist at D_2 receptors) (Figure 3.2).

▨ *1990s*: Enhanced amphetamine-induced release of DA in patients with schizophrenia compared with controls using single photon emission computerised tomography (SPECT) imaging implies presynaptic DA system abnormalities in schizophrenia (Figure 3.3).

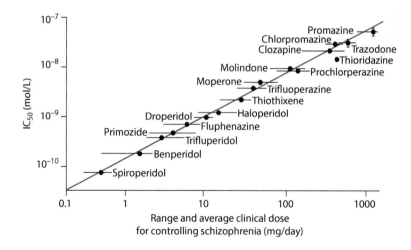

Figure 3.1 Affinity for DA receptors and clinical potency. (Reprinted by permission from Creese I et al., *Science* 1976; 192: 481. Copyright 1976, American Association for the Advancement of Science.)

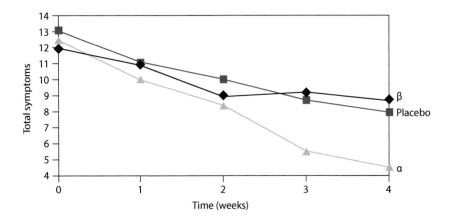

Figure 3.2 Efficacy of α- and β-flupentixol in schizophrenia. The α-isomer caused a greater improvement in symptomatology than placebo, whilst the β-isomer was without antipsychotic efficacy. (Reproduced by permission from Johnstone E et al., *Lancet* i, 1978; 848.)

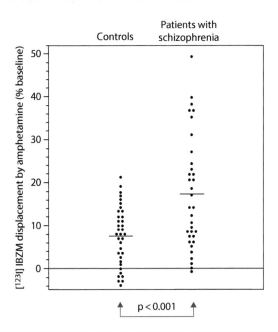

Figure 3.3 Dopamine transmission and schizophrenia. This graph illustrates the effect of amphetamine (0.3 mg/kg) on [^{123}I]IBZM binding in healthy control subjects and untreated patients with schizophrenia. The results indicate that when challenged with amphetamine, patients with schizophrenia release more dopamine than healthy controls. The amount of release is related to the increase in positive symptoms. (Reproduced by permission from Laruelle M et al., *Acad Sci USA* 1996; 93: 9235.)

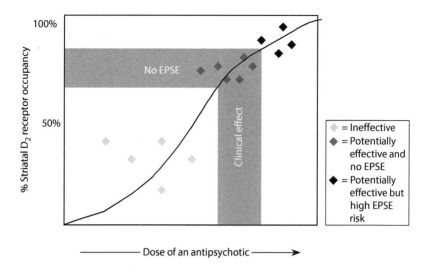

Figure 3.4 D$_2$-like receptor occupancy levels, clinical efficacy and side effects. D$_2$ receptor occupancy between 60% and 80% is associated with efficacy with minimal extrapyramidal side effects.

- *Late 1990s*: Series of neurochemical imaging experiments indicates that striatal D$_2$-like receptor occupancy above approximately 60% predicts antipsychotic efficacy, whilst greater than approximately 80%, predicts the onset of extrapyramidal side effects (EPSEs) (Figure 3.4).
- *Late 2000s*: Positron emission tomography (PET) imaging studies show that the effectiveness of antipsychotics against positive symptoms is associated with D$_2$ receptor blockade in the striatum, not with blockade elsewhere.
- *2010s*: PET studies find that mesolimbic DA is not abnormal in schizophrenia, refuting the classical DA theory. Rather, increased DA presynaptic function in the nigrostriatal pathway (particularly the part that projects to associative striatum) is associated with psychosis, and also found in people at ultra-high risk of psychosis, correlating positively with the severity of prodromal symptoms (Figure 3.5).
- *2014*: The largest genome-wide analysis of schizophrenia to date identifies more than 100 genetic regions that contribute to disease risk, including the gene for the D$_2$ receptor (DRD2; 11q23.2) and many genes involved in glutamatergic neurotransmission and synaptic plasticity.

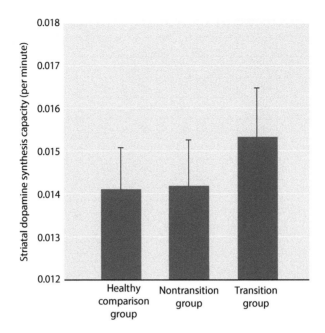

Figure 3.5 Mean DA synthesis capacity, measured by [^{18}F]DOPA PET, in patients at ultra-high risk of psychosis (n = 24) followed for 3 years and healthy comparison subjects (n = 29). Transition to first episode psychosis (n = 9) was associated with raised DA synthesis capacity in striatum at baseline compared with those who did not (n = 15). (Reprinted by permission from Howes O D et al., *Am J Psychiatry* 2011; 168: 1311.)

Role of dopamine receptor subtypes
(see also Chapter 1)

The *D_2 receptor subtype* has been the one most strongly associated with psychosis and its treatment:

- *In support*:
  - Regardless of their different psychopharmacological actions, typical and atypical antipsychotics share the property of blocking the D_2 receptors, with positive correlation between clinically effective antipsychotic dose and D_2 affinity
  - Meta-analysis of PET and SPECT imaging studies shows a small (12%) but significant increase in striatal D_2 receptor density in untreated schizophrenia, likely to reflect genetic risk
  - The D_2 receptor gene has been identified as one of the genes that contribute to the risk of developing schizophrenia

- However, this is unlikely to be the whole story as
  - About 20%–50% of patients do not respond to D_2 antagonists
  - Some atypical antipsychotics achieve an antipsychotic effect without high D_2 occupancy

The role of D_3 and D_4 receptor subtypes in schizophrenia is uncertain:

- *In support*:
  - Some atypical antipsychotics have a high affinity for D_3 and D_4 receptors
  - D_3 and D_4 receptors are distributed in proportionately higher densities in limbic areas
  - Some post-mortem studies suggested that D_3 and D_4 receptor densities in the brain may be greater in schizophrenia
- *Evidence against*:
  - The largest genome-wide study to date identified the D_2 gene as a risk factor but did not find D_3 or D_4 gene variants occurring in excess in patients with schizophrenia.
  - Unlike the D_2 receptor, there is no significant correlation between clinically effective antipsychotic dose and a drug's D_3 affinity.
  - Drugs with potent D_4 or $D_4/5-HT_{2A}$ antagonism are not antipsychotic.

Currently, the focus is moving away from the mesolimbic system as an antipsychotic drug target.

Therapeutic actions of antipsychotic drugs

- The chemical classification of older and newer antipsychotics is given in Tables 3.1 and 3.2 and their clinical uses in Table 3.3.
- Given that each of the newer antipsychotics belongs to a different chemical class, attention has turned to delineating their different pharmaceutical properties.
- Initial optimism about a general advantage of newer antipsychotics over older ones was countered by studies such as CATIE and Cost Utility of the Latest Antipsychotic Drugs in Schizophrenia Study (CUtLASS) (see Selected clinical findings section below).

Table 3.3 Clinical indications for antipsychotic drugs

Psychiatric	Non-psychiatric
Treatment of psychosis	Nausea
Treatment of mania	Anaesthesia (premedication)
Sedation/tranquillisation	Intractable hiccough
Severe anxiety	Terminal illness
Depression (some drugs)	

- Some of the historical problems with older antipsychotic drugs were due to the high doses routinely used.
- The current NICE guidelines (2014) and the BAP guidelines (2011) recommend that the choice of antipsychotic should be tailored to the individual patient, taking into account the patient's physical health and personal preference and the side-effect profile of the antipsychotic.
- Focus has moved away from an atypical–typical/conventional antipsychotic classification (or first and second generation) towards considering individual drugs, and tailoring the dose, efficacy and side-effect profile to maximise tolerability and effectiveness. Nevertheless, these terms remain prevalent.
- NICE (2014) guidelines recommend that antipsychotic medication should not be offered to people who are at risk of developing psychosis or with the aim of decreasing the risk of psychosis, or its prevention. The BAP (2011) guidelines recommend that antipsychotics for symptom relief in this situation should only be undertaken as a carefully monitored, individual patient trial, by specialist teams.

Selected clinical findings in the treatment of acute phase schizophrenia

- In the 1964 National Institutes of Mental Health study, 463 patients with acute schizophrenia were each given a 6-week trial of chlorpromazine, fluphenazine, thioridazine or placebo. Seventy percent of the patients improved on antipsychotics compared with 25% on placebo.
- A meta-analysis of placebo-controlled trials with chlorpromazine showed it was better than placebo in all 26 studies at doses over 400–500 mg/day.
- The influential Kane et al. study (1988) showed that clozapine was more effective than chlorpromazine (30% vs. 4% response) in 268 treatment-resistant patients, with improvement in both positive and negative symptoms.
- The CATIE study randomised 1432 patients with chronic schizophrenia to typical or atypical antipsychotics. Over 18 months, olanzapine was the most effective in terms of the rates of discontinuation; the efficacy of perphenazine was similar to that of quetiapine, risperidone and ziprasidone. Olanzapine was associated with greater weight gain and increases in measures of glucose and lipid metabolism, whilst perphenazine was associated with more discontinuation for EPSEs.
- The UK CUtLASS study, a pragmatic RCT in the NHS, also showed no class advantage for second-generation antipsychotics over 1 year in terms of quality of life and other measures. However, clozapine was found to be significantly more effective than the other second-generation drugs.

- A systematic review of 72 RCTs, conducted for the NICE (2009) schizophrenia guidelines, compared the efficacy of various conventional and atypical antipsychotics and found no clinically significant differences between them. The increasing placebo response rate over time complicates interpretation of multiple comparisons in meta-analyses.
- A meta-analysis of 10 long-term studies has shown that *long-acting injectable* (LAI) antipsychotics reduce the risk of relapse compared to oral antipsychotics.

Pharmacology of clinical effects of antipsychotics

- *Antipsychotic* effect (reduction of acute, positive schizophreniform symptoms (i.e. hallucinations, delusions, some aspects of thought disorder): D_2 receptor antagonism in the striatum.
- *Tranquillisation* (a reduction in agitation and aggression): DA antagonism and sedation (see next point). This effect is utilised in rapid tranquillisation (see Chapter 9).
- *Sedation*: Antihistamine and α-adrenergic blocking properties (phenothiazines are therefore very sedative).
- *Antidepressant effect* (found with some newer antipsychotics such quetiapine): $5-HT_2$ antagonism is one probable contributing mechanism; others are likely to vary between drugs, including effects at other 5-HT receptors, NA reuptake inhibition (a property of the quetiapine metabolite, norquetiapine).

Relapse prevention

- Antipsychotics protect against relapse of positive symptoms in established schizophrenia. When stopping an antipsychotic, gradual reduction in dose lengthens the time to relapse:
  - A review of 66 studies (covering 1958–1993), with follow-up of about 8 months, found the relapse rate following medication withdrawal was 53% compared with 16% in those maintained on medication.
  - A review of 22 patient cohorts, comparing gradual with abrupt discontinuation of medication, found abrupt discontinuation resulted in a cumulative relapse rate of about 46% at 6 months and 56% at 24 months; gradual reduction halved the 6-month relapse rate.
- The overall benefit of maintenance antipsychotics in *first episode psychosis* is unclear. A recent RCT found that maintenance treatment, compared with dose reduction and guided discontinuation after 6 months remission, led to less relapse in the first 18 months, but over 7-year follow-up, this benefit was lost, and in the end resulted in inferior functional and symptomatic recovery rates.

Long-acting injectables

- Administering antipsychotics in LAI form (often called depots for older antipsychotics) allows weekly or greater intervals between doses (see Chapter 2). It results in less fluctuation in plasma drug concentration and more certain medication adherence than oral administration.
- Available drugs include fluphenazine, haloperidol, flupentixol, perphenazine and zuclopenthixol (first generation) and risperidone, olanzapine, aripiprazole and paliperidone (second generation). Pipotiazine (pipothiazine) depot was withdrawn in 2014 due to a global shortage of the active ingredient, pipotiazine palmitate.
- Given the long duration of action, a small test dose should be give on initiation of an LAI, in case there is an idiosyncratic adverse reaction.
- LAIs can be perceived as a more coercive oral medication. NICE (2014) schizophrenia guidelines emphasise the importance of taking into account the service patient's preferences and attitudes towards receiving injectables, and that the same criteria are applied to the choice of LAI as to those for oral antipsychotics.

Adverse effects of antipsychotic drugs

As newer antipsychotics have become more established, the focus has shifted from the side effects common with older antipsychotics (especially EPSE) to those of the newer drugs (especially metabolic effects and weight gain).

Extrapyramidal side effects

The vast majority of extrapyramidal movement disorders seen in psychiatry are attributable to drug side effects, but they have been described in treatment naïve, first episode cases:

- Care must be taken when prescribing any antipsychotic drug, although their propensity to cause EPSE at therapeutic doses differs.
- EPSEs are generated by the blockade of D_2 receptors in the basal ganglia (see Chapter 1), specifically in the sensorimotor part of the striatum. There are four main forms of EPSE (Table 3.4).

Acute dystonia and drug-induced parkinsonism

- These effects are more likely with antipsychotics which have no intrinsic antagonism of muscarinic ACh receptors (mACh) (e.g. butyrophenones), and are less likely with antipsychotics with intrinsic mACh

Table 3.4 Extrapyramidal side effects of antipsychotics

1. *Acute dystonia*	Oculogyric crisis
	Torticollis
	Tongue protrusion
	Facial grimacing
2. *Drug-induced parkinsonism*	Muscular rigidity
	Resting tremor
	Akinesia
3. *Akathisia*	
4. *Tardive syndromes*	Dyskinesia
	Dystonia
	Akathisia

antagonism (e.g. phenothiazines). This is because of the reciprocal actions of DA and mACh systems in the basal ganglia.

- EPSEs, by definition, are also less likely with atypical antipsychotics and proposed mechanisms for this include lower D_2 binding affinity and a high 5-HT_2/DA receptor binding ratio (see mechanisms of atypicality in Atypicality and antipsychotics section).
- *Treatment of EPSE*:
  - Reduce the dose.
  - Change drug to an atypical antipsychotic less likely to cause EPSE at therapeutic doses.
  - Add a mACh antagonist (commonly referred to as 'antimuscarinic' or less precisely, 'anticholinergic' drugs), for example, procyclidine or trihexyphenidyl (benzhexol). These drugs should not be routinely co-prescribed with antipsychotics in the absence of EPSE as there is a potential for abuse and they may retard antipsychotic effects. Some studies suggest that upto 80% of patients chronically treated with antimuscarinic drugs can have the medication withdrawn without ill effect.
  - DA agonists (e.g. bromocriptine) may be used to treat persistent rigidity/akinesia, but there is a theoretical risk of aggravation of psychotic symptoms.

Akathisia

- A highly unpleasant physical and psychological restlessness.
- The precise cause is unknown and it is difficult to treat:
  - The simplest strategy is dose reduction.
  - mACh antagonists do not appear to confer benefit.
  - Benzodiazepines (diazepam) and β-blockers may be helpful.

Tardive syndromes (Table 3.5)

- These are serious, disfiguring and often permanent movement disorders.
- The most common manifestation is tardive dyskinesia (TD) (Table 3.5), but dystonia and akathisia may also be present or predominate. Most commonly, involuntary movement of the mouth or tongue is seen, although any muscle group may be affected.
- The mechanism by which TD occurs is poorly understood. Most theories focus on the disruption of D_1/D_2 receptor stimulation balance by antipsychotics, but significant incidence of dyskinesia has also been observed in untreated patients with schizophrenia.
- TD affects about 40%–50% of long-term-treated patients, usually coming on after months to years of treatment (hence tardive), but cases

Table 3.5 Features of tardive dyskinesia	
Ocular muscles	*Neck*
Blinking	Retrocollis
Blepharospasm	Torticollis
Facial	*Trunk*
Spasms	Shoulder shrugging
Tics	Pelvis rotation or thrusting
Grimaces	Diaphragmatic jerks
	Rocking
Oral	Forced retroflexion
Pouting	
Sucking	*Limbs*
Lip smacking	Finger movements
Pursing	Wrist torsion and flexion
	Arm writhing or ballismus
Masticatory	Ankle torsion and flexion
Chewing	Foot tapping
Lateral movements	Toe movements
Lingual	*Others*
Tongue protrusion	Generalised rigidity
'Fly-catching' tongue	
Writhing movements	
Pharyngeal	
Palatal movements	
Swallowing	
Abnormal sounds	

have been reported after a single episode of exposure to an antipsychotic. The incidence is highest in the first few years of treatment, with men and women equally affected.

- The risk of TD increases with age, and may occur in normal ageing without antipsychotic exposure. The emergence of TD is not predicted by the dose of antipsychotic used, or whether antimuscarinic medication has been employed.
- Available evidence suggests that newer antipsychotics have a lower risk of TD than older drugs (particularly haloperidol), but the risk is not absent. A review reported a 3% annual TD rates for newer antipsychotics compared with 7.7% for older drugs in adults.
- *Treatment of TD*:
  - If possible, the antipsychotic (and any associated antimuscarinic) medication should be gradually withdrawn or reduced: An initial exacerbation of the dyskinesia can be expected.
  - Consider clozapine as an alternative antipsychotic.
  - Consider benzodiazepines (e.g. clonazepam).
  - Consider tetrabenazine (depletes vesicular DA).
  - There are open trials of many other drugs (e.g. vitamin E), but controlled data are lacking.
  - Up to approximately 55% of patients may show recovery within a year with antipsychotic reduction or switch to clozapine.
  - Neurosurgery (pallidotomy) may be helpful in extreme cases.

Neuroleptic malignant syndrome

- A relatively rare but severe syndrome (0.5%–1% of patients) characterised by
  - Muscular rigidity
  - Decreased conscious level
  - Hyperthermia
  - Labile blood pressure
  - Increased creatinine kinase
- The disorder evolves rapidly over 24–72 h and lasts for 10–14 days if untreated. Between 5% and 20% of patients on oral medication and up to 30% of patients on depot formulations who develop the full syndrome will die from the condition if untreated. The usual cause of death is renal failure secondary to rhabdomyolysis.
- Treatment of neuroleptic malignant syndrome: The syndrome represents a serious medical emergency:
  - Antipsychotic drugs must be withdrawn immediately.
  - Dantrolene may be used to reduce muscle spasm.
  - The DA receptor agonist bromocriptine may be employed to reverse anti-DAergic effects.

- ECT, which activates DA systems, has also been used.
- Intensive care facilities may be required.
- If it is necessary to use antipsychotic medication after recovery, a 2-week interval should be observed and a structurally dissimilar antipsychotic gradually introduced with careful monitoring.

Metabolic effects and weight gain

- There has been recent concern about a link between antipsychotics, especially atypical antipsychotics, and metabolic abnormalities including diabetes and the metabolic syndrome (abdominal obesity, dyslipidemia, hypertension, insulin resistance or glucose intolerance, prothrombotic and proinflammatory states).
- The independent risk due to the drugs themselves is difficult to determine:
  - There is an increased risk of diabetes in schizophrenia itself.
  - Patients often smoke and have little regular exercise.
  - Weight gain is common. This is especially seen with clozapine and olanzapine, but a recent meta-analysis comparing 15 antipsychotics found that all except for haloperidol, lurasidone and ziprasidone caused significantly more weight gain than placebo.
  - Differences between drugs are unclear, with conflicting evidence, but clozapine and olanzapine seem to be the most likely to cause glucose dysregulation.
- When prescribing antipsychotics (especially atypicals), screening for diabetes should be considered and active management of its risk factors (e.g. weight gain) should be undertaken (see Atypicality and antipsychotics section below).

Cardiovascular and cerebrovascular events

Cardiac conduction effects

- Sudden cardiac death associated with antipsychotic use has long been recognised.
- Antipsychotic medications block the repolarisation of K^+ currents and prolong the QT interval (usually reported as QTc – corrected for heart rate), increasing the risk of ventricular tachyarrhythmias.
- The increased risk of sudden cardiac death is similar between conventional and atypical antipsychotics, and this risk is dose related in both groups. However, epidemiological and ECG studies suggest antipsychotics differ in their effects on the QT interval and their link with sudden death.

- A likely mechanism is differential blockade by antipsychotics of the delayed rectifier K$^+$ channel (I$_{Kr}$) in the myocardium, encoded for by the human ether-a-go-go (HERG) gene.
- These findings have led to lowering the maximum recommended dose of haloperidol, restrictions on the use of thioridazine and sertindole with monitoring requirements and the withdrawal of droperidol (see also Chapter 12).

Stroke

- An increased risk of cerebrovascular events has been reported in patients with dementia treated with risperidone and olanzapine, but this may also apply to other antipsychotics (see also Chapter 8).

Other adverse effects of antipsychotics (See Table 3.6)

- Many adverse effects are predictable from the receptor binding profile of the individual drugs, such as antimuscarinic symptoms, sedation, postural hypotension and to some extent weight gain. Other side effects are more idiosyncratic.

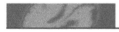 **Monitoring patients on antipsychotics**

The 2014 NICE schizophrenia guidelines give recommendations for monitoring that should be carried out for patients prescribed antipsychotics:

- Before starting an antipsychotic,
  - Determine the weight, waist circumference, pulse and blood pressure, fasting blood glucose (FBC), glycosylated haemoglobin (HbA1c), blood lipid profile and prolactin levels and assess for presence of movement disorders (also assess diet, nutritional status and physical activity)
  - Perform ECG if indicated by cardiovascular risk or specific drug requirements
- After starting drug treatment,
  - Monitor weight and for EPSE emergence regularly especially early in treatment and when titrating
  - At 3 months, determine the weight, EPSE, pulse and blood pressure, FBC, HbA1c and blood lipids
  - Annually: As at 3 months + waist circumference

Table 3.6 Non-extrapyramidal adverse effects of antipsychotic drugs

Antimuscarinic (due to potent M_1 receptor antagonism)	Dry mouth and sore throat. Constipation. Blurred near vision. Tachycardia. Urinary retention. Abuse potential. Acute confusion in overdose.
Anti-adrenergic (due to potent α_1 and α_2 receptor antagonism)	Postural hypotension and reflex tachycardia. Small pupils.
Sedation	Contributed to by H_1 and α-adrenergic antagonism (especially clozapine, chlorpromazine, ziprasidone and quetiapine).
Cardiotoxicity	Contributed to by delayed conduction, M_1 antagonism and α-adrenergic antagonism. Slowing of cardiac conduction time (increased QTc) leading to sudden death (especially thioridazine, pimozide). Possibility of causing myocarditis has been raised.
Hepatotoxicity	Chronically raised liver enzymes.
Impaired glucose tolerance/diabetes mellitus	Especially clozapine, olanzapine, but many others. NB increased baseline risk in schizophrenia.
Weight gain	Predicted by a drug's antagonist potency at H_1, 5-HT_{2A}, 5-HT_{2C}, M_3, α_1 and α_2 receptors. Also due to drug's effects on leptins. Especially clozapine, olanzapine, iloperidone, chlorpromazine.
Hyperprolactinaemia (predicted by potent D_2 receptor antagonism)	Caused by D_2 receptor antagonism in the tuberoinfundibular pathway at the top of the pituitary stalk. Conventional and some atypical antipsychotics such as risperidone, paliperidone and amisulpride.
Blood dyscrasias	Well known with clozapine, but shared by all antipsychotics to a lesser extent.
Photosensitivity	Especially chlorpromazine; use sun block.

Atypicality and antipsychotics

- The problem of EPSEs with 'typical' antipsychotics, and the increased efficacy of clozapine compared with other antipsychotics, has encouraged the search for 'atypical' clozapine-like drugs without its drawbacks.
- The distinction between 'typical' and 'atypical' is not clear (some prefer the terms 'older' and 'newer' or 'first generation' and 'second generation'), and these terms are now seen to have little discrimination when referring to classes of drugs.
- It is more meaningful to consider drugs individually, each having more or less 'atypicality'.

Definitions of atypicality

- A number of factors have been proposed to define 'atypicality' compared with older, 'typical' or conventional, antipsychotics:
  - Greater efficacy for positive symptoms
  - Greater efficacy for negative symptoms
  - Lower tendency to cause EPSE
  - Failure to increase serum prolactin
- However, the most parsimonious definitions are related to decreased tendency to cause EPSE:
  - *Pre-clinically*: A clinically effective antipsychotic that does not produce catalepsy in rats
  - *Clinically*: A drug with wide therapeutic ratio such that EPSE are not seen at clinically effective antipsychotic doses
- The therapeutic range can be conceptualised as lying between two doses of any antipsychotic:
  - A lower dose at which, in a group of patients, 50% will achieve some clinical benefit; this is the minimum effective dose.
  - An upper dose at which 50% of the group of patients will experience some form of mild EPSE.
  - The older, typical, antipsychotics generally had a very narrow dose range, roughly equating to 6–7 mg of haloperidol equivalents. Newer, atypical, antipsychotics generally have a wider range, allowing one to predict a dose which is likely to be effective but unlikely to cause EPSE.

Mechanisms of atypicality

Atypical antipsychotics vary in their pharmacological properties. It is likely that a number of mechanisms confer different aspects of atypicality:

- *Reduced EPSE*:
  - Lower D_2 affinity
  - High $5\text{-HT}_2/D_2$ binding ratio

- – Limbic selective D_2 receptor antagonism
- – D_2 receptor partial agonism
- – mAChR antagonism (NB high levels of M_1 antagonism may exacerbate psychosis)
- ▨ *Reduced hyperprolactinaemia*:
  - – Lower D_2 affinity
  - – D_2 receptor partial agonism
- ▨ Increased efficacy against negative symptoms; proposed mechanisms include
  - – Pre- versus post-synaptic D_2 antagonism
  - – 5-HT_2 antagonism
  - – D_2 receptor partial agonism
  - – Absence of EPSE simulating a beneficial effect on negative symptoms

Clozapine (described in detail in the next section) represents the prototypical atypical antipsychotic, illustrating the features described earlier:

- ▨ Low incidence of EPSE
- ▨ Does not stimulate prolactin secretion
- ▨ Effective in treatment-resistant cases
- ▨ Improves negative as well as positive symptoms
- ▨ High affinity for M_1 receptor with relatively low affinity for D_2 receptor
- ▨ D_2 limbic selectivity

Distribution of pharmacological mechanisms amongst atypical drugs

- ▨ High affinity for cholinergic M_1 receptors: Clozapine and olanzapine
- ▨ Lower affinity for striatal D_2 receptors: Clozapine, quetiapine and olanzapine
- ▨ Higher affinity for 5-HT_{2A} receptors than for striatal D_2 receptors: Risperidone, sertindole, ziprasidone, olanzapine, clozapine and quetiapine
- ▨ Higher affinity for limbic D_2 and D_2-like receptors than for striatal D_2 receptors: Clozapine, sertindole, amisulpride, quetiapine and risperidone (any limbic selectivity is lost at higher doses for all, except possibly clozapine)
- ▨ D_2 receptor partial agonism: Aripiprazole

Individual newer/atypical antipsychotics (listed alphabetically)

- ▨ Drugs are licensed for the treatment of psychosis/schizophrenia in the United Kingdom and United States unless otherwise stated. Where relevant, specific licences are detailed, but for full information including marketing authorisations, consult the relevant national summary of product characteristics.

- In the United Kingdom, zotepine was the latest antipsychotic drug to be withdrawn (in 2011), although still available in some countries, and lurasidone the most recently introduced (2014).
- Drugs currently in development include brexpiprazole (related to aripiprazole) and cariprazine (a $D_3 > D_2$ partial agonist).
- There are a number of drugs licensed in the Far East that are not available in the United States or United Kingdom/EU (blonanserin, nemonapride, perospirone). Melperone, available in a number of EU countries but not the United Kingdom or United States, is related to haloperidol, but has a low affinity for D_2 receptors and an 'atypical' adverse-effect profile.
- A recent multiple-treatment meta-analysis compared the efficacy and tolerability of 15 antipsychotics. Efficacy results are shown in Figure 3.6:
  - Most drugs have similar efficacy; clozapine is the most effective followed by amisulpride, olanzapine and risperidone.

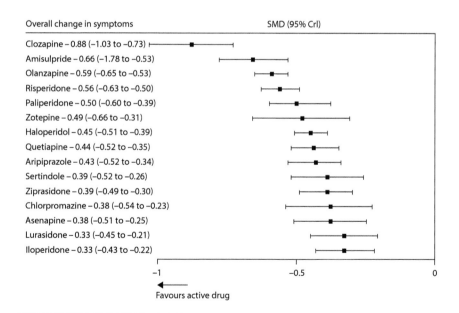

Figure 3.6 Forest plot from a multiple-treatment meta-analysis of the efficacy of antipsychotic drugs compared with placebo. SMD, standardised mean difference; CrI, credible interval. (Reproduced by permission from Leucht S et al., *Lancet* 2013; 382: 951.)

- Rankings for different adverse effects (e.g. EPSE, weight gain) are mainly as predicted from their pharmacology and clinical profile (see the following list). QTc prolongation is greatest for sertindole, amisulpride and ziprasidone and least for lurasidone, aripiprazole and paliperidone; all cause discontinuation is highest with haloperidol, sertindole and lurasidone and lowest for amisulpride, olanzapine and clozapine.

Amisulpride

■ Not licensed in the United States

Pharmacology

■ Selective and equipotent antagonism at D_2 and D_3 receptors
■ Limbic selective
■ Antagonist at the 5-HT_7 receptor
■ Chemically and clinically similar to sulpiride but with better absorption

Efficacy/clinical use

■ As efficacious as haloperidol for acute and chronic schizophrenia.
■ At lower doses, effective for patients with mainly negative symptoms.
■ A Cochrane review found amisulpride to be of some benefit in the treatment of dysthymia but not major depression (MDD).

Side effects

■ Low EPSE similar to placebo at lower doses
■ Less weight gain than risperidone or olanzapine
■ Dose-dependent EPSE and prolactinaemia at higher doses

Aripiprazole

■ Also licensed in the United States for augmentation of antidepressants in MDD patients with suboptimal response to antidepressant monotherapy

Pharmacology

■ Receptor binding profile: $D_2 > 5\text{-HT}_{2A} \approx 5\text{-HT}_{1A} > \alpha_1 \approx H_1 > \alpha_2 > 5\text{-HT}_{2C}$
■ High affinity D_2 receptor partial agonist
■ Acts functionally as a D_2 antagonist under most physiological conditions, but may act as D_2 agonist in prefrontal cortex where endogenous DA is potentially low in schizophrenia

- Partial agonist at 5-HT$_{1A}$ receptor
- High-affinity antagonist at 5-HT$_{2A}$ receptor
- Low-/moderate-affinity antagonist at H$_1$ and α$_1$ receptors
- No anticholinergic effect

Efficacy/clinical use

- As effective as haloperidol for acute and chronic schizophrenia
- Short-acting injectable effective for the control of agitation and behavioural disturbance in schizophrenia
- Effective in the treatment and prevention of mania
- Has antidepressant properties
- Available in LAI form (requires oral supplementation for 14 days at initiation)

Side effects

- Low EPSE similar to placebo at all doses (initial akathisia can occur in the first 2 weeks of treatment)
- Does not increase plasma prolactin levels (and may decrease levels)
- Less weight gain than most antipsychotics
- QTc changes not different to placebo

Asenapine

- Licensed in the United Kingdom and EU only for acute mania in bipolar I disorder and licensed in the United States and Australia for acute mania or mixed episodes in bipolar I disorder and for schizophrenia

Pharmacology

- Antagonist with high affinity for 5-HT$_{1A}$, 5-HT$_{1B}$, 5-HT$_{2A}$, 5-HT$_{2B}$, 5-HT$_{2C}$, 5-HT$_{5A}$, 5-HT$_6$ and 5-HT$_7$ receptors; α$_1$, α$_{2A}$, α$_{2B}$ and α$_{2C}$ adrenoceptors; D$_1$–D$_4$ receptors; and H$_1$ and H$_2$ receptors
- Low affinity for M$_1$ receptors
- Partial agonist at the 5-HT$_{1A}$ receptors
- Needs to be administered sublingually

Efficacy/clinical use

- Similar efficacy to chlorpromazine in the treatment of schizophrenia
- Appears less efficacious than risperidone and olanzapine in the treatment of acute mania

Side effects

- EPSE lower than haloperidol but higher than most other atypicals
- Low potential for elevating prolactin levels
- Less weight gain than most atypicals; similar to that of aripiprazole

Clozapine

- Clozapine is licensed for patients unresponsive to, or intolerant of, other antipsychotic drugs
- Blood monitoring and registration with monitoring service are mandatory

Pharmacology

- Receptor binding affinity profile: $H_1 \approx M_1 \approx \alpha_1 > 5\text{-HT}_{2A} > 5\text{-HT}_{2c} > \alpha_2 > D_2$ receptors
- Lower doses required in the elderly, females and non-smokers
- Metabolised to norclozapine. The clozapine/norclozapine ratio (normal average = 1.33 across dose range) may be helpful in assessing recent compliance: Ratio > 3 suggests blood drawn was not a trough sample; ratio < 0.5 suggests poor compliance in preceding days
- Hypersalivation possibly due to M_4 agonism, α_2 antagonism and inhibition of swallowing reflex

Efficacy/clinical use

- Most effective antipsychotic and treatment of choice in refractory schizophrenia: Reduces or eliminates positive symptoms in ~60% of patients resistant to other antipsychotics
- Effective for psychosis without exacerbating motor symptoms in Parkinson's disease patients who become psychotic due to dopaminergic drugs
- Aim for plasma level of at least 350 µg/L to ensure an adequate trial, but response can occur at lower levels
- Used in refractory bipolar disorder (on the basis of open data only)

Side effects/interactions

- High H_1 and α_1 affinities cause marked sedation and postural hypotension, so low initial dose and slow titration is necessary
- Risk of agranulocytosis, seizures, myocarditis and cardiomyopathy higher than other antipsychotics
- Nocturnal enuresis is common (though under-reported), particularly in early treatment
- Hypersalivation

- Avoid concomitant use with
  - Drugs that can cause agranulocytosis, for example carbamazepine, chloramphenicol and cytotoxics
  - Benzodiazepines (serious adverse effects reported)
  - Depot antipsychotics (cannot withdraw quickly if neutropenia occurs)
- Caution if used with other antimuscarinic drugs; beware of paralytic ileus and gastroparesis
- Plasma levels of clozapine increased by concomitant use of some SSRIs, possibly valproate (decreases also possible with valproate)
- Concomitant lithium can increase neutrophil and total white cell count (unlicensed indication) but caution required due to risk of EPSE and neurotoxicity. Should only be used if prior episodes of neutropenia were unrelated to clozapine

Iloperidone

- Licensed in the United States for the treatment of schizophrenia, not in the United Kingdom/EU

Pharmacology

- Structurally similar to risperidone
- Broad range of receptor antagonism: $\alpha_1 >$ 5-HT$_{2A} \approx$ D$_2 \approx$ D$_3 >$ 5-HT$_{2C} \approx \alpha_2 >$ H$_1$
- Low H$_1$ and negligible M$_1$ affinity
- Plasma levels not affected by food or smoking
- Metabolised in the liver via CYP2D6 and CYP3A4
- One of the two primary metabolites crosses the blood–brain barrier and has a similar receptor binding profile

Efficacy/clinical use

- Significantly more effective than placebo, but a network meta-analysis found its efficacy to be the lowest ranked of available second-generation antipsychotics

Side effects

- Low levels of sedation, raised prolactin and EPSE
- Initial orthostatic hypotension and dizziness significant, so start with low dose and gradual titration
- Moderate risk of QTc prolongation and weight gain
- Reduce total daily dose by 50% if used in the presence of strong CYP2D6 or 3A4 inhibitors

Lurasidone

- Also licensed for the treatment of depression in bipolar I disorder in the United States

Pharmacology

- Antagonist at α_1, α_{2A} and α_{2C} receptors; D_1 and D_2 receptors; and 5-HT$_{2A}$, 5-HT$_{2C}$ and 5-HT$_7$ receptors
- Partial 5-HT$_1$ agonist
- Recommended to be taken with food

Efficacy/clinical use

- One of the lowest ranked antipsychotics for efficacy in the treatment of schizophrenia in a network meta-analysis
- Found to be superior in reversing dizocilpine-induced learning and memory impairment compared with haloperidol, clozapine, risperidone, olanzapine, quetiapine and aripiprazole in rat studies, and may have a place in treating the cognitive and memory deficits in schizophrenia
- Acute treatment of bipolar depression

Side effects

- EPSE more likely than most atypicals, and akathisia a common side effect
- Less weight gain compared with other atypical antipsychotics; similar to ziprasidone and haloperidol
- Less QTc prolongation than most atypical antipsychotics

Olanzapine

- Also licensed for mania and maintence treatment of bipolar disorder, and in the United States for bipolar depression in combination with fluoxetine

Pharmacology

- Related to clozapine
- Broad range of receptor antagonism: $H_1 \approx M_1 \approx$ 5-HT$_{2A}$ > 5-HT$_{2C}$ > D_2 > α_1 > α_2 > D_1
- Some D_2 limbic selectivity
- Plasma levels reduced by smoking
- For the same daily dose of olanzapine, plasma levels in women are approximately 80% higher than in men

Efficacy/clinical use

- As effective as haloperidol for positive symptoms of schizophrenia
- Some evidence of better efficacy against negative symptoms of schizophrenia
- Better than risperidone for mood symptoms in schizophrenia
- Effective in the acute treatment of mania and maintenance treatment of bipolar disorder, plus in combination with fluoxetine for bipolar depression
- Short-acting injectable form available and effective for the control of agitation and behavioural disturbance
- LAI form available; post-injection monitoring required for rare post-injection syndrome (ranging from mild sedation to coma and delirium, EPSE, hypertension and convulsions)

Side effects

- EPSE = placebo in clinical doses
- Sedation
- More weight gain than most other antipsychotics
- Dizziness
- Antimuscarinic effects (dry mouth, constipation)
- Less increase in prolactin than haloperidol or risperidone
- Possible glucose dysregulation
- Post-injection syndrome

Paliperidone

Pharmacology

- The main hepatic (CYP2D6-mediated) metabolite of risperidone (9-OH-risperidone)
- Receptor antagonist profile similar to risperidone: $5\text{-}HT_{2A} > D_2 \approx \alpha_1 > 5\text{-}HT_{2C} \approx H_1 > \alpha_2$
- Less affinity for D_4 receptor than risperidone
- Bioavailability (28%) is less than risperidone (70%), so clinically equivalent dose is approximately twice the dose of risperidone
- Approximately 60% of the dose is excreted unchanged in the urine; minimal further hepatic metabolism, so potentially useful for patients with hepatic failure, high or low CYP2D6 metabolism, CYP-based drug interactions
- Available as an oral and a LAI: Smaller needle gauge and smaller injection volume compared with risperidone LAI

Efficacy/clinical use

- As efficacious as olanzapine in the treatment of schizophrenia

Side effects

- EPSE more severe than most other atypical antipsychotics
- Along with risperidone, produces the largest increases in prolactin levels compared with other antipsychotics
- Weight gain moderate; more weight gain than haloperidol, ziprasidone, lurasidone, aripiprazole and amisulpride
- QTc changes not different to placebo

Quetiapine

- Also licensed for bipolar disorder and as adjunctive treatment for depressive disorder following suboptimal response to SSRI antidepressants

Pharmacology

- Some structural resemblance to olanzapine and clozapine
- Broad range of receptor antagonism: $H_1 > \alpha_1 > 5\text{-HT}_{2A} > D_2 > 5\text{-HT}_{2C} > \alpha_2$
- D_2 limbic selectivity
- Its key metabolite, N-desalkylquetiapine (norquetiapine), is an NA reuptake inhibitor
- Short plasma half-life (7 h) of non-modified release preparations
- Plasma levels not affected by smoking

Efficacy/clinical use

- As effective as haloperidol and chlorpromazine for schizophrenia
- Possible efficacy for negative symptoms
- Effective in bipolar disorder for the treatment of mania, depression and in prophylaxis
- Effective antidepressant in MDD, both as monotherapy and adjunctive treatment

Side effects

- EPSE = placebo
- No increase in prolactin
- Sedation
- Dizziness
- Constipation
- Less frequent – dry mouth, weight gain

Risperidone

- Licensed for mania in bipolar I disorder; in the United Kingdom, licensed for short-term treatment in moderate-to-severe Alzheimer's dementia and for persistent aggression in conduct disorder and in the United States, licensed for the treatment of irritability in autistic children and adolescents

Pharmacology

- Receptor antagonism: $5\text{-HT}_{2A} > D_2 \approx \alpha_1 > 5\text{-HT}_{2C} \approx H_1 > \alpha_2$
- Low/moderate histamine H_1 affinity
- Minimal antimuscarinic, D_1, 5-HT_1 affinity
- D_2 limbic selective only at lower doses
- Available as LAI (requires oral supplementation for 21 days after the first injection)

Efficacy/clinical use

- Large number of positive multicentre RCTs in schizophrenia
- Possible bell-shaped dose–response curve
- Uncertain if effective for negative symptoms
- Effective in the acute treatment of mania and continuation of treatment in bipolar disorder (including naturalistic data for the LAI formulation)

Side effects

- Less drug-induced parkinsonism than typical antipsychotics at lower doses, but dystonias and akathisia can occur
- Tachycardia
- Some weight gain
- Hyperprolactinaemia can be pronounced

Sertindole

- Withdrawn due to concerns about increase in QTc; limited reintroduction in 2002 in Europe under strict ECG monitoring regimen

Pharmacology

- Receptor antagonism: $5\text{-HT}_{2A} > \alpha_1 > D_2$-family $(D_2 \approx D_3 \approx D_4)$
- D_2 limbic selectivity

Efficacy/clinical use

- Effective against positive and negative symptoms of schizophrenia

Side effects

- EPSE = placebo
- Weight gain – comparable to quetiapine
- Minimal short-term increase in prolactin
- Increase in QTc – needs ECG monitoring
- Nasal congestion, decreased ejaculatory volume, postural hypotension and dry mouth
- Occasionally raised liver enzymes

Ziprasidone

- Licensed in the United States for the treatment of schizophrenia and bipolar I disorder and parts of Europe; not in the United Kingdom

Pharmacology

- Receptor antagonism: $5\text{-}HT_{2A} > D_2 \approx 5\text{-}HT_{2C} > \alpha_1 > H_1 > \alpha_2$
- Possible limbic selective D_2 antagonism
- Weak $5\text{-}HT_{1A}$ receptor partial agonism
- Negligible antimuscarinic effect
- Weak 5-HT and NA reuptake inhibition

Efficacy/clinical use

- Perhaps slightly more effective than haloperidol
- Possible efficacy for negative symptoms of schizophrenia
- Possible efficacy for depressive symptoms in schizophrenia
- Effective in the acute treatment of mania or mixed episodes

Side effects

- EPSE = placebo
- No appreciable weight gain
- Headache, nausea and insomnia are the most common side effects (but <10% of patients)
- Insomnia, pharyngitis, rash and tremor are more common than with placebo
- Increases QTc

Acknowledgement

This is an update and revision of the third edition chapter by Michael Travis and Ian C Reid.

 **Bibliography**

Guidelines

Barnes T and the Schizophrenia Consensus Group of the British Association for Psychopharmacology. Evidence-based guidelines for the pharmacological treatment of schizophrenia: Recommendations from the British Association for Psychopharmacology. *J Psychopharmacol.* 2011; 25: 567–620. http://bap.org.uk/pdfs/Schizophrenia_Consensus_Guideline_Document.pdf.

De Hert M, Dekker JM, Wood D et al. Cardiovascular disease and diabetes in people with severe mental illness: Position statement from the European Psychiatric Association (EPA), supported by the European Association for the Study of Diabetes (EASD) and the European Society of Cardiology (ESC). *Eur Psychiat.* 2009; 24: 412–424.

National Institute for Health and Care Excellence. Psychosis and schizophrenia in adults: Treatment and management. *NICE Clinical Guideline 178.* 2014; http://www.nice.org.uk/guidance/cg178.

Key references

Agid O, Mamo D, Ginovart N et al. Striatal vs extrastriatal dopamine D2 receptors in antipsychotic response—A double-blind PET study in schizophrenia. *Neuro Psychopharmacol.* 2007; 32: 1209–1215.

Bollini P, Pampallona S, Orza MJ et al. Antipsychotic drugs: Is more worse? A meta-analysis of the published randomised controlled trials. *Psychol Med.* 1994; 24: 307–316.

Creese I, Burt DR, Snyder SH. Dopamine receptor binding predicts clinical and pharmacological potencies of antischizophrenic drugs. *Science.* 1976; 192: 481–483.

Cunningham-Owens DG. Adverse effects of antipsychotic agents. Do newer agents offer advantages? *Drugs.* 1996; 51: 895–930.

Geddes J, Freemantle N, Harrison P, Bebbington P. Atypical antipsychotics in the treatment of schizophrenia: Systematic overview and meta-regression analysis. *BMJ.* 2000; 321: 1371–1376.

Howes OD, Bose SK, Turkheimer F et al. Dopamine synthesis capacity before onset of psychosis: A prospective [18F]-DOPA PET imaging study. *Am J Psychiatry.* 2011; 168: 1311–1317.

Johnstone E, Crow TJ, Frith CD et al. Mechanism of the antipsychotic effect in the treatment of schizophrenia. *Lancet.* 1978; i: 848–851.

Jones PB, Barnes TR, Davies L et al. Randomized controlled trial of the effect on Quality of Life of second- vs first-generation antipsychotic drugs in schizophrenia: Cost Utility of the Latest Antipsychotic Drugs in Schizophrenia Study (CUtLASS 1). *Arch Gen Psychiatry.* 2006; 63: 1079–1087.

Kane J, Honigfeld G, Singer J, Meltzer H. Clozapine for the treatment-resistant schizophrenic: A double-blind comparison with chlorpromazine. *Arch Gen Psychiatry.* 1988; 45: 789–796.

Leucht C, Heres S, Kane JM et al. Oral versus depot antipsychotic drugs for schizophrenia—A critical systematic review and meta-analysis of randomised long-term trials. *Schizophr Res.* 2011; 127: 83–92.

Leucht S, Cipriani A, Spineli L et al. Comparative efficacy and tolerability of 15 anti-psychotic drugs in schizophrenia: A multiple-treatments meta-analysis. *Lancet.* 2013; 382(9896): 951–962.

Lieberman JA, Stroup TS, McEvoy JP et al. Clinical Antipsychotic Trials of Intervention Effectiveness (CATIE) Investigators. Effectiveness of antipsychotic drugs in patients with chronic schizophrenia. *N Engl J Med.* 2005; 353: 1209–1223.

Schizophrenia Working Group of the Psychiatric Genomics Consortium. *Nature.* 2014; 511: 421–427.

Further reading

Correll CU, Schenk EM. Tardive dyskinesia and new antipsychotics. *Curr Opin Psychiatry.* 2008; 21: 151–156.

De Hert M, Detraux J, van Winkel R et al. Metabolic and cardiovascular adverse effects associated with antipsychotic drugs. *Nat Rev Endocrinol.* 2011; 8: 114–126.

Haddad P, Dursun S, Deakin B. *Adverse Syndromes and Psychiatric Drugs: A Clinical Guide.* Oxford, UK: Oxford University Press, 2004.

Hegarty JD, Baldessarini RJ, Tohen M et al. One hundred years of schizophrenia: Meta-analysis of the outcome literature. *Am J Psychiatry.* 1994; 151: 1409–1416.

Hirvonen J, van Erp TGM, Huttunen J et al. Increased caudate dopamine D2 receptor availability as a genetic marker for schizophrenia. *Arch Gen Psychiatry.* 2005; 62: 371–378.

Laruelle M, Abi-Dargham A, van Dyck CH et al. Single photon emission computerized tomography imaging of amphetamine-induced dopamine release in drug-free schizophrenic subjects. *Proc Natl Acad Sci USA.* 1996; 93: 9235–9240.

Ray WA, Chung CP, Murray KT et al. Atypical antipsychotic drugs and the risk of sudden cardiac death. *N Engl J Med.* 15, 2009; 360: 225–235.

Seeman P. Atypical antipsychotics: Mechanism of action. *Can J Psychiatry.* 2002; 47: 27–38.

Stahl S. *Essential Psychopharmacology: Neuroscientific Basis and Practical Implications*, 4th edn. Cambridge, UK: Cambridge University Press, 2013.

Taylor D. Low-dose typical antipsychotics—A brief evaluation. *Psychiatr Bull.* 2000; 24: 465–468.

Taylor D, Paton C, Kapur S. *The Maudsley Prescribing Guidelines in Psychiatry*, 12th edn. 2012 John Wiley & Sons Ltd.: Chichester, UK, 2015.

Urban N, Abi-Dargham A. Neurochemical imaging in schizophrenia. *Curr Top Behav Neurosci.* 2010; 4: 215–242.

Wheeler AL, Voineskos AN. A review of structural neuroimaging in schizophrenia: From connectivity to connectomics. *Front Hum Neurosci.* 2014; 8: 653.

Antidepressants and ECT

Chris Smart, Ian M Anderson and
R Hamish McAllister-Williams

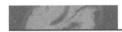 ## History

The first effective antidepressant agents of the modern era were discovered by chance in the late 1950s:

- Iproniazid (monoamine oxidase inhibitor [MAOI]): Developed originally as an antitubercular drug.
- Imipramine (tricyclic antidepressant [TCA]): Developed originally as a chlorpromazine analogue (by Kuhn in 1957).
- MAOIs and tricyclics have the common property of interacting with monoamine systems – dopamine (DA), noradrenaline (NA) and serotonin (5-HT).

Monoamine hypothesis of depression

The monoamine hypothesis was originally proposed in the 1960s based on the actions of drugs. Monoamine promoters relieved depression, while the monoamine-depleting drug reserpine led to depressive symptoms.

- Schildkraut – Proposed catecholamines (NA, DA) to be functionally deficient in depression and elevated in activity in mania.
- Ashcroft – Proposed indolamines (5-HT) to be functionally deficient in depression. This led to the development of 5-HT-selective drugs in the 1970s and subsequently the selective serotonin reuptake inhibitors (SSRIs).
- The monoamine hypothesis has been greatly modified over subsequent decades with the focus moving from neurotransmitter turnover to receptor regulation and second messenger signalling.
- A current hypothesis proposes a common pathway for antidepressant action involving increased 5-HT neurotransmission, via altered

receptor sensitivity, leading to increased activation of cortical 5-HT$_{1A}$ postsynaptic receptors.

- SSRIs, for example, block serotonin reuptake leading to increased 5-HT in the raphe nucleus. This initially increases activation of somatodendritic 5-HT$_{1A}$ autoreceptors on raphe serotonergic neurons leading to decreased neural firing and hence 5-HT release. However over time, the 5-HT$_{1A}$ autoreceptors are desensitised/downregulated restoring neuronal firing and, in the presence of ongoing reuptake blockade, there is increased synaptic 5-HT and activation of postsynaptic 5-HT$_{1A}$ receptors (Figure 4.1).
- The hypothesis does not explain satisfactorily the similarity in efficacy of very different agents acting differentially on monoamine systems.
- The action of antidepressants on monoamine neurotransmission does not of itself mean that these systems are abnormal in depression.
- Furthermore, evidence for primary monoamine disturbance in depressed subjects is limited and somewhat inconsistent, as outlined in the next sections.

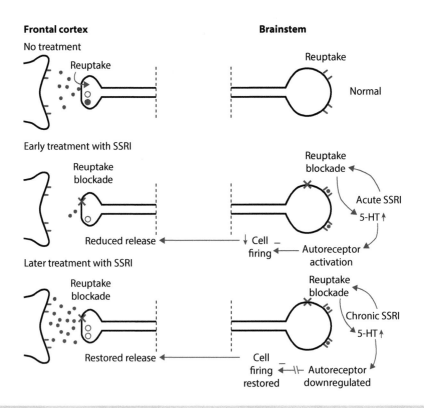

Figure 4.1   Current 5-HT hypothesis of how antidepressant drugs work.

Serotonin

▦ Reduced 5-HT metabolites in the cerebrospinal fluid (CSF) of depressed subjects as well as in post-mortem brain tissue of those who have committed suicide.

▦ Increased platelet/brain 5-HT_2 receptor binding sites in depressed patients.

▦ Downregulation of postsynaptic 5-HT_{1A} receptors in depressed subjects. Corroborated by neuroendocrine studies: Decreased prolactin response to tryptophan infusion and reduced buspirone-induced hypothermia; positron emission tomography (PET) studies showing reduced brain 5-HT_{1A} receptor binding.

▦ Relapse of depression induced by tryptophan depletion in SSRI-treated and drug-free recovered depressed patients.

Noradrenaline

▦ Reduced levels of the CNS NA metabolite, 3-methoxy-4-hydroxyphenylglycol (MHPG), in urine of depressed subjects.

▦ Possible postsynaptic α_2-receptor downregulation in depression. Neuroendocrine studies show reduced growth hormone response to the α_2-agonist clonidine and insulin-induced hypoglycaemia.

▦ Decreased responses to β-receptor agonists in depression.

▦ Relapse of depression induced by α-methyl paratyrosine (NA synthesis inhibitor) in patients treated with NA reuptake inhibitors (NARIs).

Dopamine

▦ Increased D_2 receptor numbers in some PET studies of depressed patients.

▦ Mood-elevating effects of DA-releasing psychostimulants.

▦ Possible antipsychotic-induced depression (high dose – postsynaptic DA receptor blockade).

▦ Possible antipsychotic antidepressant activity (low dose – presynaptic DA autoreceptor blockade leading to feedback dysregulation and increased DA release).

▦ Preclinical studies consistently implicate DA systems in neural basis of reward (related to anhedonia).

 ## Other hypothesised pathophysiological mechanisms

▦ Given the shortcomings of the monoamine hypotheses to fully explain the pathophysiology of depression and its treatment, hypotheses concerned with alternative neurobiological systems have been proposed.

- Two prominent areas of research have concerned the hypothalamic–pituitary–adrenal (HPA), or stress, axis, and mechanisms related to neuroplasticity.
- There has also been recent interest in inflammation as a contributory factor.
- Hypotheses of abnormalities in different neurobiological systems are not mutually exclusive (or with monoamine systems) as they interact and are all involved in emotional processing.

HPA axis

- HPA axis abnormalities are implicated in, but not specific to, nor ubiquitous in, depressive disorder.
- Complex interactions between 5-HT and corticosteroid systems in system CNS may account for the relationship between the stress and cognitive dysfunction in depressive disorder.
- Many depressed patients exhibit elevated cortisol levels and non-suppression of cortisol in the 'dexamethasone suppression test'.
- Toxic effects of dysregulated cortisol may lead to degenerative changes (e.g. reduced hippocampal volume) seen in depressive disorder and neuroplasticity abnormalities (see next section).
- Adverse early experience – physical, emotional or sexual abuse – may alter HPA axis function in a long-lasting way, conferring vulnerability to depression and stress-related disorders in adulthood.
- However, treatment trials (as monotherapy and augmentation of monoamine antidepressants) of agents influencing the HPA axis have produced inconsistent results. These include glucocorticoid receptor antagonists (e.g. mifepristone), cortisol synthesis inhibitors (e.g. metyrapone), corticotropin-releasing hormone antagonists and vasopressin V1b antagonists.

Glutamate and neuroplasticity hypotheses (Figure 4.2)

- Recent research indicates that in depressive disorder there is a reduction in neuroplasticity and upregulation of the excitatory neurotransmitter glutamate.
- Monoamines are thought to act through second messenger signalling (e.g. mitogen-activated protein kinase, MAPK and cAMP) that in turn alter gene transcription and culminate in normalised neuroplasticity and glutamate levels.
- Drugs that directly target excess glutamate have been shown to have rapid effects on synaptogenesis and improve mood (e.g. ketamine), though effects are not prolonged.

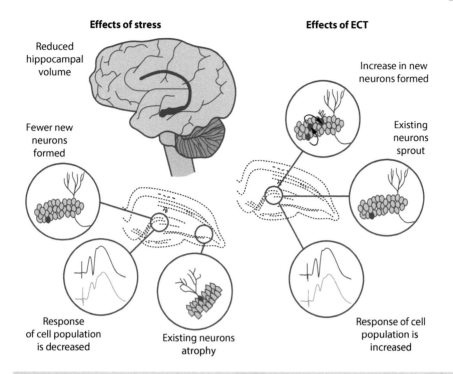

Effects of stress

Reduced hippocampal volume

Fewer new neurons formed

Response of cell population is decreased

Existing neurons atrophy

Effects of ECT

Increase in new neurons formed

Existing neurons sprout

Response of cell population is increased

Figure 4.2 Reciprocal effects of stress and ECT on neurons. (Courtesy of Dr CA Stewart, University of Dundee, Dundee, United Kingdom.)

▦ Intriguingly, antidepressant agents, including electroconvulsive therapy (ECT), have common cellular effects leading to enhanced expression of neuroprotective proteins (e.g. BDNF) that bolster neuronal survival and regulate synaptic connectivity.
  – In rats, antidepressant medication and ECT promote cell production in the dentate gyrus of the hippocampus and possibly reversing the toxic effects of HPA axis abnormalities (Figure 4.2).
  – Preliminary studies in some stress-related disorders, such as post-traumatic stress disorder, suggest that antidepressant drugs can reverse volumetric abnormalities in limbic system structures such as hippocampus.
▦ However, as yet there is no treatment specifically directed at glutamate and/or neuroplasticity (except possibly ECT) in routine clinical use.

Emotional processing

▦ Depression is associated with a negative cognitive bias – i.e., patients have a tendency to preferentially focus on negative stimuli, or to recall negative memories, compared to positive ones.

- Antidepressants have been shown to have direct effects on emotional processing, including after single doses in healthy subjects; either a reduction in negative bias or an increase in positive bias depending on the drug.
- Changes in emotional processing early during treatment with an antidepressant have been found to predict therapeutic response.

Antidepressant drugs

- At the present time, all antidepressants in routine clinical use have prominent, usually primary, effects on monoamine neurotransmission (Figure 4.3).
- Traditional methods of grouping antidepressants are confusing, at times defining drugs on the basis of the pharmacology (e.g. SSRIs) and at times on the basis of structure (e.g. TCAs).
- Marketing approval varies between countries; the drugs described later are licenced in the United States and the United Kingdom except where stated.
- Only the major available antidepressants available in the United Kingdom and/or the United States are described.

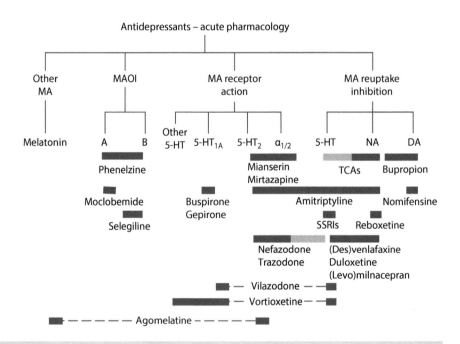

Figure 4.3 Acute pharmacology of some antidepressants.

Selective serotonin reuptake inhibitors (SSRIs)

SSRIs are the most common first-line antidepressant used for depression and anxiety disorders.

Neurochemistry

- All share the property of relatively selective 5-HT reuptake blockade but are structurally distinct.
- Most have some minor degree of other actions on different neurotransmitter systems.

Pharmacokinetics

- Rapidly absorbed.
- Hepatically metabolised – may be affected by individual cytochrome P450 (CYP450, CYP) enzyme differences.
- Some have active metabolites (Table 4.1).
- Low concentrations in breast milk (highest levels with fluoxetine/citalopram, lowest with sertraline/paroxetine).
- Discontinuation syndrome (see below) possible with short half-life drugs (paroxetine most likely, fluoxetine least).

Efficacy

- Little evidence for dose–response in usual dose range (except possibly escitalopram 10 and 20 mg); dose titration not required.

Table 4.1 Selective comparative pharmacology of SSRIs

	Active metabolite	$T_{1/2}$ – h (active metabolite)	Cytochrome P450 inhibition (isoenzyme)
Citalopram	–	36	–
Escitalopram (S-enantiomer of citalopram)	–	36	–
Fluoxetine	+++	72 (200)	+++ (2D6, 3A4, 2C19)
Fluvoxamine	–	15	++ (1A2, 2C19)
Paroxetine	–	20	+++ (2D6, 2C9)
Sertraline	+	25 (66)	+ (2D6)

- Useful in the elderly, comorbid anxiety/obsessive-compulsive disorder (OCD), suicidal patients (safer in overdose than TCAs).
- Escitalopram (*S*-enantiomer of citalopram) may be more effective than citalopram. This is attributed to escitalopram binding to both the reuptake (orthosteric) site and an allosteric site causing conformational change in the 5-HT transporter and enhancing reuptake blockade. *R*-enantiomer of citalopram blocks this conformational change. This is not seen with other SSRIs.

Side effects

- *Gastrointestinal (GI) effects*: Nausea (most common), vomiting, diarrhoea, constipation (activation of postsynaptic 5-HT$_3$ receptors).
- *Sedation/dizziness* in 10%–20%.
- *Sexual dysfunction* common in males and females (possibly activation of postsynaptic 5-HT$_2$ receptors). Appears most prominent with paroxetine, least with escitalopram/fluvoxamine.
- *Hyponatraemia* (biggest risk in elderly) due to syndrome of inappropriate anti-diuretic hormone (SIADH) secretion.
- Increased *risk of bleeding* (due to depletion of platelet 5-HT). Gastroprotective agents recommended in those at risk of GI bleed.
- Citalopram and escitalopram associated with a dose-dependent *increase in QTc* on ECG.
- *Agitation*.
- *Movement disorders*.
- *Parkinsonism* (uncommon).
- *Convulsions* (rare).

Interactions

Useful interactions:

- TCAs, lithium, L-tryptophan (but caution warranted)

Problematic interactions:

- MAOIs, L-tryptophan and St John's wort can lead to serotonin syndrome if prescribed with SSRIs (see Serotonin sydrome section).
- SSRIs can inhibit CYP2D6 and CYP3A3/4 and increase levels of antipsychotics, opiates and TCAs.
- Fluvoxamine can inhibit CYP1A2 and increase levels of clozapine, theophylline and caffeine.

Serotonin and noradrenaline reuptake inhibitors (SNRIs)

Also known as 'dual action' reuptake inhibitors, and include venlafaxine, duloxetine and milnacipran (the latter not available in the United States/ the United Kingdom but is prescribed in France and Japan, and its active enantiomer, levomilnacipran is in clinic development). They are often used in depressed patients failing to respond to an SSRI. Venlafaxine has been associated with an increased risk of manic switch in bipolar depression.

Venlafaxine

- Selective 5-HT and NARI (NA reuptake inhibition only when dose above 150 mg/day). DA reuptake inhibition may occur at higher doses. These effects at different doses may explain an apparent dose–response relationship when treating depression which is not seen with SSRIs.
- May have enhanced efficacy in severe depressive disorder at higher doses.
- Dose-dependent increase in blood pressure, needs regular monitoring at higher doses ($\geq$300 mg/day).
- Can increase risk of seizures, especially in overdose.
- Can cause prominent discontinuation syndrome (similar symptoms to SSRIs).
- Other side effects essentially similar to SSRIs. At higher doses it causes additional side effects related to NA effects including dry mouth, urinary retention, blurred vision and constipation. Sweating is a common side effect, especially at higher doses.

Desvenlafaxine

- This is the major metabolite of venlafaxine (*O*-desmethylvenlafaxine) licenced in North America, but not in the European Union (apart from Spain).
- It has a greater NA:5-HT transporter inhibition ratio than venlafaxine.
- It has little hepatic metabolism with a lower risk of pharmacokinetic interaction than venlafaxine.
- It is well tolerated at the recommended dose, but side effects similar to venlafaxine occur at higher doses without increased efficacy.

Duloxetine

- Selective 5-HT and NARI (affinity for both transporters similar).

- Like other drugs blocking both 5-HT and NA reuptake (e.g. venlafaxine and amitriptyline), it has efficacy in treating neuropathic and musculoskeletal pain.
- Potential to cause/exacerbate liver disease, hence, should not be used with alcohol.
- Side effects as for venlafaxine. Also associated with fatigue.

Serotonin reuptake inhibitors with additional pharmacological actions

This is a heterogeneous group of drugs; some have been in use for a number of years (e.g. trazodone) while others are newer (vilazodone and vortioxetine).

Phenylpiperazines

Licenced examples are trazodone and nefazodone.

- Relatively weak 5-HT reuptake inhibition.
- $5-HT_2$ antagonist properties which may have antidepressant and anxiolytic properties as well as reducing the impact of serotonin reuptake on sexual dysfunction.
- Other pharmacological actions include $5-HT_{1A}$ partial agonism, α_1 antagonism and weak H_1 antagonism (trazodone). m-Chlorophenylpiperazine is a metabolite with 5-HT agonist properties and may have antidepressant action.
- Relatively safe in overdose.
- Side effects include GI upset, sedation (especially trazodone), headache, dizziness and hypotension (rarely priapism with trazodone).
- Nefazodone was withdrawn from Europe in 2003 due to hepatotoxicity; use is subject to monitoring of hepatic function in the United States.

Vortioxetine

- Novel mechanism of $5-HT_3$ (as well as $5-HT_{1D/7}$ to lesser degree) antagonism, $5-HT_1$ agonism and $5-HT_{1B}$ partial agonism in addition to 5-HT reuptake inhibition.
- Increases 5-HT, NA, DA as well as cholinergic, histaminergic, GABAergic and glutamatergic action in preclinical models.
- Effects localised to dorsal and median raphe nuclei and the prefrontal cortex.
- Side effects include nausea, dizziness and sexual dysfunction at higher doses.

- Reported to cause less cognitive impairment and possibly improve cognition.
- National Institute for Health and Care Excellence (NICE) appraisal scheduled for 2015.

Vilazodone

- This is licenced in the United States, but not in the European Union.
- 5-HT reuptake inhibitor and partial agonist at somatodendritic 5-HT_{1A} autoreceptors.
- Claims that leads to a more rapid downregulation of 5-HT_{1A} autoreceptors and, thus, more rapid onset of therapeutic action.
- Well tolerated. Side effects include GI upset and insomnia. Sexual dysfunction similar to placebo.
- Comparability to other antidepressants uncertain at present.

(Selective) noradrenaline reuptake inhibitors (NARIs)

Current available drugs are reboxetine and the TCA lofepramine. These are licensed in the European Union, but not in the United States.

- Relatively specific reuptake inhibitors of NA. Increase NA transmission as well as DA in prefrontal cortex.
- Efficacy may be less than SSRIs and serotonin and noradrenaline reuptake inhibitors (SNRIs).
- May have alerting properties.
- Side effects include insomnia, postural hypotension, sweating and anticholinergic-like side effects, probably due to functional interaction between sympathetic and parasympathetic nervous systems.
- Lofepramine is a TCA (its major metabolite is desipramine), but it is included here as it differs from other TCAs by lacking significant toxicity in overdose and low affinity for monoamine receptors.

Noradrenaline and dopamine reuptake inhibitors

The only example available at present is amfebutamone (more commonly called bupropion). Licenced in the United States for depression, but not in the United Kingdom where licence is as an adjunct for smoking cessation (see Chapter 7).

- It is unrelated in structure to other antidepressants. Exact mechanism of action remains uncertain.
- Has anticraving properties and can cause weight loss.

- Side effects include dry mouth, insomnia, anxiety, GI upset, sweating, hypertension and at higher doses may cause seizures (contraindicated in epilepsy as well as eating disorders, alcohol withdrawal and recent head injury where there is also an increased risk of seizures).
- Low apparent risk of causing switching to mania in bipolar disorder (as also seen with SSRIs).
- Used in combination with SSRIs in the United States for treatment-resistant depression, sexual dysfunction and apathy.

α_2-Adrenoceptor antagonists

Mirtazapine and mianserin

- Mirtazapine is an α_2-adrenergic, 5-HT$_2$, 5-HT$_3$ and H$_1$ antagonist.
- Mianserin is a much older drug and is not licenced in the United States, and its mechanism of action is not fully clear. It shares most of mirtazapine's pharmacology but also antagonises α_1-adrenergic receptors and may inhibit reuptake of NA.
- Mirtazapine is relatively sedative (H$_1$ antagonism), which may be less at higher doses (possibly due to NA stimulation).
- Both drugs activate NA neurons by blocking the negative feedback of NA on presynaptic α_2-adrenoceptors.
- Increased noradrenergic activity stimulates 5-HT neuron activity in the brainstem (via α_1-adrenoceptors), while blockade of α_2-adrenoceptors on 5-HT terminals in the cortex also enhances 5-HT release.
- Net effect is to increase activity in both NA and 5-HT systems; the effect on 5-HT may be stronger with mirtazapine which lacks α_1-antagonism.
- Blockade of 5-HT$_2$ and 5-HT$_3$ (mirtazapine only) receptors thought to minimise sexual dysfunction and nausea, respectively, and may be related to low likelihood of side effects.
- Side effects include sedation, weight gain, abnormal dreams and blood dyscrasia (the latter is more common with mianserin and blood count needs monitoring).
- Can be combined safely with SSRIs and SNRIs (most commonly mirtazapine is used for this) in treatment refractory patients. Well tolerated due to 5-HT$_2$ and 5-HT$_3$ receptor blockade, reducing side effects of SSRIs and SNRIs.

Tricyclic antidepressants (TCAs)

This is a pharmacologically heterogeneous group of drugs.

- Their primary therapeutic pharmacological action may be similar to an SSRI (e.g. clomipramine), an SNRI (e.g. amitriptyline) or a NARI (e.g. lofepramine, desipramine). As metabolites of tertiary amines are

NARIs (see later text), it is best to consider TCAs as NARIs with a variable amount of 5-HT reuptake inhibition.

▪ A few TCAs have negligible monoamine reuptake inhibition (e.g. trimipramine).

▪ They have been retained as a class here due to some commonality in relation to their other pharmacological affects contributing to their side effect profile and contraindications.

Neurochemistry

▪ 5-HT reuptake inhibition and/or NA reuptake inhibition.

▪ Tertiary amines are generally more potent 5-HT reuptake blockers (but are metabolised to secondary amines).

▪ Secondary amines are more potent at blocking NA reuptake.

▪ Receptor antagonism varies widely between drugs from considerable (e.g. amitriptyline with α_1-adrenoceptor, 5-HT_2, M_1, H_1 antagonism) to minimal (e.g., desipramine).

▪ Most are Na^+ and L-type Ca^{2+} channel blockers.

Pharmacokinetics

▪ Rapidly absorbed and widely distributed.

▪ Hepatically metabolised: May be influenced by individual CYP2D6 metaboliser status.

▪ Tertiary amines are metabolised to secondary amines, for example amitriptyline to nortriptyline and imipramine and lofepramine to desipramine (desmethylimipramine).

▪ Selected comparative pharmacology of some TCAs is shown in Table 4.2.

Table 4.2 Selective comparative pharmacology of TCAs

Drug (active metabolite)	$T_{1/2}$ – h (active metabolite)	NA uptake inhibition	5-HT uptake inhibition	Anticho- linergic	Sedation
Amitriptyline (nortriptyline)	16 (36)	++	+++	+++	+++
Imipramine (desipramine)	16 (24)	++	+++	++	++
Clomipramine (desmethylclomipramine)	18 (36)	+	+++	++	+
Nortriptyline	36	+++	+	++	+
Dosulepin (northiaden)	20 (40)	+	+	++	++
Lofepramine (desipramine)	5 (24)	+++	+	+	+

Efficacy

- Some evidence for differential dose–response and its side effects are dose-related; therefore, there is need to titrate to effective doses.
- Increasingly used more often for inpatients, where potential side effects can be monitored more easily.
- Side effects, and cardiac toxicity, also mean they are less commonly used in the elderly, the physically ill and those with a history of suicide.

Side effects

- *Anticholinergic*: Dry mouth, blurred vision, constipation, urinary retention.
- *Antihistaminergic*: Sedation, weight gain.
- α_1-*Adrenoceptor blockade*: Postural hypotension, dizziness, sedation.
- *5-HT_2 blockade*: Weight gain (especially amitriptyline).
- *Cardiotoxic (Na^+ and Ca^{2+} channel blockade)*: QTc prolongation, arrhythmias and possibly ST elevation.
- *Neurotoxic*: Delirium, movement disorders, seizures, coma.
- *Discontinuation syndrome*: General somatic symptoms, insomnia, vivid dreams, GI symptoms, mood symptoms including anxiety, agitation and rarely psychosis.
- *Manic switch*: In bipolar patients – probably enhancement of NA neurotransmission.

Interactions

Useful interactions

- Lithium, L-tryptophan (but caution warranted).

Problematic interactions

- SSRIs (especially fluoxetine, paroxetine) may inhibit TCA metabolism leading to higher TCA plasma levels.
- MAOIs may lead to serotonin syndrome especially clomipramine with tranylcypromine.
- Alcohol potentiates TCA sedation.
- Cimetidine increases TCA levels.
- Warfarin potentiated or inhibited by different TCAs.
- Phenothiazines and haloperidol may increase TCA levels.

Contraindications

- Heart block and other arrhythmias
- Recent myocardial infarction
- Hypomanic or manic phase of bipolar affective disorder
- Acute porphyria

Monoamine oxidase inhibitors (MAOIs)

The risk of adverse reactions with older MAOIs has relegated them to specialist use after failure to respond to other drugs. Moclobemide is not licenced in the United States, and transdermal selegiline is not licenced in the European Union/the United Kingdom.

Neurochemistry

- MAO is present peripherally, especially the gut, as well as the CNS.
- MAO-A metabolises NA, 5-HT, DA and tyramine. MAO-B metabolises DA, tyramine and phenylethylamine.
- Traditional MAOIs inhibit both MAOI-A and MAO-B.
- MAOIs increase storage and release of 5-HT and NA.
- Traditional MAOIs (phenelzine, tranylcypromine, isocarboxazid) and some relatively selective MAO-B inhibitors (e.g. selegiline) produce irreversible inhibition, and restoration of function needs synthesis of new enzymes.
- Moclobemide is a reversible inhibitor of MAO-A (RIMA); the potential for interaction with tyramine/indirect sympathomimetics is greatly reduced as the drug is displaced from the enzyme.

Pharmacokinetics

- Rapid absorption on oral administration.
- Toxic levels can occur in slow acetylators.
- Transdermal administration (with selegiline) reduces GI effects and first-pass metabolism, so the need for food restrictions and the risk of hypertensive crises are much less.
- Half-life is less important than time taken to replace stores of MAO after irreversible blockade, and at least 2 weeks is needed before switching to a new antidepressant that could interact (e.g. SSRI, SNRI).
- Moclobemide has a short half-life and this, together with its reversibility, means that no washout period is needed when switching to a new antidepressant.

Efficacy

- Traditional MAOIs are third-line treatment but retain an important place in therapy. Clinically they tend to be used in the following situations (but high-quality evidence is lacking):
  - Severe depression, especially with lethargy and poor motivation.
  - Depression resistant to treatment; may also be combined with lithium and/or L-tryptophan.

- – Atypical depression – Presence of mood reactivity, excessive sleep and weight gain, sensitivity to rejection as a personality trait (*DSM-IV/5*).
- – Anxiety disorders resistant to other treatments (see also Chapter 6).
- Moclobemide is well tolerated and does not require specialist supervision. It had good efficacy in randomised controlled trials (RCTs) but clinical experience has been less positive, possibly because of underdosing (use its maximum licenced dose).
- Experience with transdermal selegiline is limited.

Side effects

- These mostly apply to traditional MAOIs and include
  - – Nausea, dizziness, restlessness, sweating, tremor, insomnia, sexual difficulties
  - – Postural hypotension (especially in the elderly)
  - – Peripheral oedema (especially phenelzine)
- Tranylcypromine appears more stimulant than phenelzine, but with fewer other side effects. It has been associated with abuse and dependence.
- Hypertensive reaction (see below)

Interactions

- *Sympathomimetics*: Hypertensive reaction (see next section). Moclobemide has very limited potential for this because of its selectivity for MAO-A and its reversible mode of action; transdermal selegiline because of relative selectivity for MAO-B and route of administration.
- *Other antidepressants*: Combination with SSRIs, SNRIs or serotonergic TCAs (clomipramine) can cause the serotonin syndrome (see earlier section).
- *Pethidine*: Respiratory depression, CNS excitation or depression.
- *Alcohol, barbiturates*: CNS depression.
- *Insulin*: Impaired blood glucose control.
- *Antiepileptics*: Lower seizure threshold.

Hypertensive reaction/crisis

- *Causes*:
  - – Tyramine-containing foods (dietary tyramine is normally inactivated in the gut by MAO), e.g. cheese, yeast extracts, hung game, certain alcoholic drinks, broad bean pods and pickled herring
  - – Indirect sympathomimetic drugs such as phenylephrine (e.g. non-prescription cold remedies)

- *Symptoms*:
  - Flushing
  - Headache (typically back of head)
  - Increased blood pressure
  - Cerebrovascular accident (rare)
- *Management*:
  - *Prevention*: Education, food warning leaflets.
  - *Treatment*: α-Adrenergic blockade with phentolamine or phenoxy-benzamine; chlorpromazine is a useful alternative if these are not available (and a small stock can be kept by the patient).

Contraindications

- Cardiovascular or cerebrovascular disease
- Phaeochromocytoma
- Hyperthyroidism
- Hepatic disease
- Delirium

Other antidepressants

Agomelatine

- Agomelatine is licenced in the European Union/the United Kingdom, but not in the United States.
- Efficacy appears equal to other antidepressants in clinical trials but less established in clinical practice.
- It is an agonist at melatonin MT_1 and MT_2 receptors and an antagonist of $5\text{-}HT_{2C}$ receptors.
- Its mechanism of action is uncertain, but is reported to increase DA and NA in prefrontal cortex.
- Side effects include nausea, dizziness, sedation and GI upset, but these are rare. This is due to the drug being taken at night with a half-life of around 1.5 h; hence, there are negligible blood levels during the day.
- Raised liver enzymes (up to 2.5% of patients at higher dose) and hepatotoxicity (rare) mean LFT monitoring are required.

Other drugs with antidepressant properties

- *Newer (atypical) antipsychotics* (see Chapter 3 for details)
  - Evidence for efficacy as an adjunctive treatment with antidepressants (especially SSRIs) for quetiapine, aripiprazole, risperidone and, to a lesser extent, olanzapine.
  - Quetiapine is also effective as monotherapy.

- Lower doses needed than when used as an antipsychotic.
- Mechanism of antidepressant action not clear and may differ between drugs; candidates include 5-HT$_2$ antagonism, NA reuptake inhibition (quetiapine metabolite) and DAergic effects.

- *Lithium* (see Chapter 5 for details)
  - Effective as an adjunctive treatment to antidepressants (most evidence with TCAs).
  - Use has decreased with the availability of new drugs, the complexities of its use and adverse effects (see Chapter 5).
  - The mechanism of antidepressant action includes enhancing 5-HT function.

- *L-Tryptophan*
  - Precursor of 5-HT.
  - Weak antidepressant. Primarily used as an adjunct with MAOIs and TCAs.
  - Withdrawn from United Kingdom market as a prescription drug but available as food supplement.
  - Possible side effects include sedation, headache, myoclonus and serotonergic syndrome (when used in combination with other serotonergic drug).
  - Eosinophilia–myalgia syndrome previously described due to a contaminated Japanese batch of drug. No longer seen as a risk.
  - Sudden discontinuation in patients who respond can lead to rapid (within 24 h) return of depressive symptom.

- *S-Adenosylmethionine*
  - Available as a prescription drug in some European Union countries (not the United Kingdom) and as food supplement in the United States and the United Kingdom.
  - Evidence for antidepressant efficacy given orally and intravenously.
  - Well tolerated, but includes reports of GI symptoms, insomnia and serotonin syndrome in combination with serotonergic drugs.
  - Acts as a methyl donor in metabolic reactions involved in cellular growth and repair and neurotransmitter and hormone synthesis.

- *St John's wort (Hypericum perforatum)*
  - Available as herbal product in the European Union and the United States. Popular in German-speaking countries.
  - Active ingredients include hypericin and hyperforin but many other potential plant substances are also present. Mechanism of action believed to be due to inhibition of monoamine reuptake, especially 5-HT.
  - Systematic reviews show efficacy, especially in mild depression, with less certainty in more severe major depression.
  - Well tolerated, but side effects include nausea, vomiting, constipation, sedation and dizziness and increased risk of serotonin syndrome with other serotonergic agents.

- – Induces CYP3A4 and risk of interactions with many drugs including antiarrhythmics, anticoagulants, Ca^{2+} channel blockers and cytotoxics and can also reduce plasma levels of amitriptyline.
- – Not recommended in NICE (2009) guidance for the treatment of depression.
- *Ketamine*
  - – It is a dissociative anaesthetic with analgesic properties.
  - – It is an antagonist at glutamate NMDA receptors.
  - – RCTs have show it to have a rapid antidepressant action (within hours) when given intravenously, but its benefit is not maintained unless re-administered.
  - – Its adverse effects (dissociative phenomena and longer term potential for haemorrhagic cystitis, colitis and hepatitis and abuse) and route of administration make it an experimental treatment, but there is interest in developing safer oral glutamatergic drugs.
- *Anti-inflammatory drugs*
  - – A recent meta-analysis found that anti-inflammatory drugs used alone reduced depressive symptoms in physical illness (most studies were in osteoarthritis), with a moderate effect size.
  - – In four small short-term RCTs in major depression, celecoxib (a selective COX-2 inhibitor) had a small to moderate benefit over placebo when combined with an SSRI/NARI.
  - – It is not known whether anti-inflammatories are only of use in individuals with demonstrably raised inflammatory cytokines nor the appropriate duration of treatment.

Specific adverse effects of antidepressants

Antidepressant discontinuation syndrome

The occurrence of this syndrome has led to claims that antidepressants are 'addictive'. While indicating physiological adaptation to the drug has occurred, other aspects of the addiction (such as craving, tolerance, dose escalation) are not seen (although rarely described with tranylcypromine which has amphetamine-like properties).

- *Symptoms*:
  - – Usually begin within 3–5 days of abruptly stopping established (i.e. for a number of weeks) treatment with antidepressants, particularly those with short half-lives.
  - – Are variable and differ between classes of antidepressants, but include sleep disturbance and increased dreams, GI symptoms, mood disturbance (including mania), EPSE and general somatic symptoms (such as lethargy and headache) and rarely psychosis.
  - – Have been particularly associated with some SSRIs (especially paroxetine and venlafaxine) where additional prominent symptoms

include sensory abnormalities (including electric shock-like sensations, paraesthesia and disequilibrium/dizziness).
- MAOIs may cause more severe symptoms including confusion and psychotic symptoms.
- *Management*:
  - Usually mild and self-limiting over 1–2 weeks.
  - Education and reassurance usually sufficient.
  - If more severe, restart antidepressant and taper more slowly; for SSRIs/SNRIs, consider switch to/start fluoxetine (because of long half-life), and then withdraw the drug.

Serotonin syndrome

- This is an acute neuropsychiatric condition due to increased CNS 5-HT activity (when severe it can be confused with neuroleptic malignant syndrome).
- It has been described with a wide range of drugs, not just SSRIs and SNRIs.
- Mild forms may be overlooked and put down to side effects of restlessness or agitation; severe forms need urgent management.
- It is rarely an idiosyncratic reaction to a serotonergic drug but is usually due to pharmacodynamic interactions between drugs that enhance 5-HT function (e.g. SSRI + MAOI).
- Symptoms include confusion, myoclonic jerks, hyperreflexia, pyrexia, sweating, autonomic instability, GI symptoms and mood change including mania.
- Management is based on stopping the offending drug/s and supportive measures; symptoms usually subside rapidly.

Suicidality

- There has been concern that some antidepressants, particularly SSRIs, might cause *increased suicidality* in some patients.
- Suicidal acts are predominantly due to depression itself. They are most common before treatment starts and decrease through the early treatment period.
- Current consensus is that antidepressants (not just SSRIs), compared with placebo, slightly increase the risk of suicidal ideation or suicidal behaviour in adolescents and younger adults up to age of 25 years (although risk of completed suicide has not been demonstrated) but have a neutral or protective effect in older adults which increases with age. Population studies have tended to find that antidepressant use is associated with decreased suicide rates.

- The UK Committee on Safety of Medicines (2003) declared that only fluoxetine had a favourable risk–benefit ratio in adolescents. The US Food and Drug Administration has issued a 'black box' warning for increased suicide risk with the use of antidepressants in children and young adults.
- All patients need to be monitored for suicidal risk during treatment, with particular care taken with younger patients.

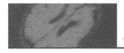 ## Using antidepressants effectively (see also Chapter 11)

- Antidepressant efficacy is best established for moderate to severe unipolar major depression and chronic depression of any severity.
- The efficacy of antidepressants in bipolar depression is controversial and first-line treatment is mood stabilisers and/or atypical antipsychotics. If antidepressants are used, they should always be combined with an antimanic agent (see Chapter 5). SSRIs appear less likely to cause manic switch than drugs with NA reuptake inhibition.
- Ensure that adequate doses are used (TCAs need titrating) and alter initial treatment if needed between 3 and 6 weeks if there is inadequate response.
- There is little to choose between antidepressants in terms of efficacy for initial treatment: Adverse effect profile and previous treatment experience are the main considerations.
- SSRIs are considered first-line antidepressants. A network meta-analysis of 12 newer generation antidepressants found the following:
  - *Highest ranked for efficacy* were mirtazapine, escitalopram, venlafaxine and sertraline.
  - *Highest ranked for tolerability* (discontinuation of treatment) were escitalopram, bupropion, sertraline and citalopram.
  - *Lowest ranked for efficacy and tolerability* were reboxetine, duloxetine, fluvoxamine and milnacipran.
- Treatment of non-response includes switching antidepressants, addition of psychological treatment, adjunctive agents (especially an atypical antipsychotic or lithium) and ECT.
- Effective prophylaxis is vital following remission; at least 6–12 months if the risk of relapse is low and longer (sometimes indefinitely) for recurrent depression or partial remission.
- Decreasing to a maintenance dose is an obsolete concept: 'The dose that gets you better keeps you better'.

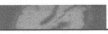 ## Electroconvulsive therapy

Although not a psychopharmacological treatment, ECT is briefly considered here because of evidence for similar effects to antidepressant drugs and its role in the treatment of severe depression.

History

- ECT has its roots in the mistaken idea that schizophrenia and epilepsy were mutually exclusive conditions.
- Convulsions were initially induced chemically; in the 1930s safer, electrical induction of seizures was developed (Cerletti and Binet).
- Initially, 'unmodified' ECT was used (i.e. without muscle relaxant); from the 1950s, general anaesthesia and muscle relaxation have employed to reduce the risk of fractures during a seizure.
- Large open trials in the 1960s and blinded, randomised placebo-controlled trials in the 1970s and 1980s demonstrated the acute efficacy of ECT in depressive disorder.
- It remains one of the most effective, yet controversial treatments in medicine, the latter partly due to its portrayal in the media, but due also to professional attacks related to its adverse effects and lack of RCT evidence for long-term benefit.
- The use of ECT is decreasing. This may be due in part to more systematic and effective treatments for depressive disorder, but also due to greater difficulty accessing it with less frequent inpatient treatment, and loss of professional confidence and experience. The impact of patients being denied such an effective treatment remains unclear.

Mode of action

- ECT results in a generalised tonic–clonic seizure from electricity applied either across the brain (bilateral) or across one hemisphere (right unilateral in a right-handed person). Repeated administrations are needed to produce its antidepressant, and antipsychotic, effect (twice weekly in the United Kingdom, three times weekly in the United States).
- The mode of action of ECT, like chemical antidepressant therapy, is poorly understood but appears to depend on both the dose of electricity and achieving an adequate seizure.
- Similar effects to antidepressant medication upon monoamine systems have been described; DA systems may be particularly affected.
- Electroconvulsive stimulation has been shown to have neuroprotective effects and stimulates neurogenesis in preclinical models.

- ECT is a potent anticonvulsant and may share properties with some mood-stabilising agents.
- There is no convincing evidence that ECT as given in usual clinical practice causes significant brain damage.

Indications

- Evidence for efficacy is strongest in depressed patients with psychosis and psychomotor retardation. ECT tends to be reserved for situations where
  - Alternative treatments have failed
  - A rapid response is necessary in the face of intense suicidality
  - Dangerous self-neglect or inanition
  - Intractable psychotic depressive states
- NICE guidance in the United Kingdom (2003, 2009) recommends its use for the acute treatment of moderate and severe depression, mania or catatonia only in patients who have failed to respond to other treatments; it is not recommended in schizophrenia.

Outcome/efficacy

- ECT appears to be extremely acutely effective in depression, with a remission rate greater than that of drug or psychological treatment (typically 50%–80%), including in patients who have failed to respond to previous treatments. Patients receiving ECT represent a more severe and 'treatment-resistant' population than those receiving other treatments.
- Efficacy and cognitive side effects appear related to the dose of current applied.
- A direct comparison of matched patients (with random allocation) has not been made with contemporary antidepressant or psychological care.
- Relapse rates are high (especially in treatment-resistant patients), with 50% or more of patients relapsing within the year following treatment.
- Continuation/maintenance ECT appears effective in depressed patients who relapse after successful treatment with ECT but evidence to support it is thin.

Side effects

- The principal physical hazards of ECT lie with those adverse events encountered in general following brief general anaesthesia. It is recommended that senior anaesthetists experienced in the use of ECT conduct sessions.
- Headache and nausea are common and respond to conventional treatment.

Cognitive impairment

- It can be difficult to disentangle the cognitive effects of ECT from those of depression itself, where it tends to improve concurrently with mood.
- Cognitive impairment is related to method of administration (bilateral > unilateral, possibly because the left hemisphere speech centres are spared), stimulation parameters (sine wave > brief pulse), electrical dose and patient-specific factors (age, cognitive reserve, cerebrovascular disease).
- The following main types are described:
  - *Acute confusion*: Disorientation immediately following treatment typically lasting for about 20 min.
  - *Anterograde amnesia and executive function deficits*: These develop during the course of ECT but can be demonstrated early in the treatment. They resolve within a few weeks of stopping ECT, and repeated courses of ECT or maintenance treatment do not lead to cumulative lasting impairment.
  - *Retrograde amnesia*: Lack of memory for events during the ECT course is not uncommon related to anterograde amnesia. Loss of past memories, particularly autobiographical memories, is variable but can be very distressing for some patients. Objective demonstration of its frequency and severity and understanding the phenomenon have been hampered by lack of adequate research tools. For some, it may improve with time but is experienced as permanent by others.

Cautions and contraindications

Absolute

- Raised intracranial pressure
- Recent cerebrovascular accident
- Unstable vascular aneurysm
- Recent myocardial infarction with unstable rhythm

Relative

- Pregnancy
- Retinal detachment
- Cerebral tumour
- History of cerebrovascular accident

Acknowledgement

This is an update and revision of the third edition chapter by Ian C Reid.

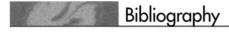 **Bibliography**

Guidelines

Cleare A, Pariante CM, Young AH et al. Evidence-based guidelines for treating depressive disorders with antidepressants: A revision of the 2008 British Association for Psychopharmacology guidelines, *J Psychopharmacol.* 2015; 29: 459–525. http://bap.org.uk/pdfs/antidepressants.pdf.

National Institute for Health and Care Excellence. Depression in adults: The treatment and management of depression in adults. *Nice Clinical Guideline 90.* 2009; http://www.nice.org.uk/Guidance/CG90 (this also updates the ECT guidance for depression only).

National Institute for Health and Care Excellence. Depression in adults with a chronic physical health problem: Treatment and management. *Nice Clinical Guideline 90.* 2009; http://www.nice.org.uk/guidance/CG91.

National Institute for Health and Care Excellence. Guidance on the use of electroconvulsive therapy. *NICE Technology Appraisal Guidance 59.* 2003; http://www.nice.org.uk/guidance/TA59 (NB ECT for depression updated in NICE CG90).

Key references

Anderson IM. Selective serotonin reuptake inhibitors versus tricyclic antidepressants: A meta-analysis of efficacy and tolerability. *J Affect Disord.* 2000; 58: 19–36.

Cipriani A, Furukawa TA, Salanti G et al. Comparative efficacy and acceptability of 12 new-generation antidepressants: A multiple-treatments meta-analysis. *Lancet.* 2009; 373(9665): 746–758.

Gartlehner G, Hansen RA, Morgan LC et al. Comparative benefits and harms of second-generation antidepressants for treating major depressive disorder: An updated meta-analysis. *Ann Intern Med.* 2011; 155: 772–785.

Geddes JR (for the UK ECT review group). Efficacy and safety of electroconvulsive therapy in depressive disorders: A systematic review and meta-analysis. *Lancet.* 2003; 361: 799–808.

Geddes JR, Carney SM, Davies C et al. Relapse prevention with antidepressant drug treatment in depressive disorders: A systematic review. *Lancet.* 2003; 361(9358): 653–661.

Harmer CJ, Goodwin GM, Cowen PJ. Why do antidepressants take so long to work? A cognitive neuropsychological model of antidepressant drug action. *Br J Psychiatry.* 2009; 195: 102–108.

Moller HJ, Bitter I, Bobes J et al. Position statement of the European Psychiatric Association (EPA) on the value of antidepressants in the treatment of unipolar depression. *Eur Psychiatry.* 2012; 27: 114–128.

Reid IC, Stewart CA. How antidepressants work. *Br J Psychiatry.* 2001; 178: 299–303.

Renoir T. Selective serotonin reuptake inhibitor antidepressant treatment discontinuation syndrome: A review of the clinical evidence and the possible mechanisms involved. *Front Pharmacol.* 2013; 4: 45.

Rush AJ, Trivedi MH, Wisniewski SR et al. Acute and longer-term outcomes in depressed outpatients requiring one or several treatment steps: A STAR*D report. *Am J Psychiatry.* 2006; 16: 1905–1917.

Spielmans GI, Berman MI, Linardatos E et al. Adjunctive atypical antipsychotic treatment for major depressive disorder: A meta-analysis of depression, quality of life, and safety outcomes. *PLoS Med.* 2013; 10: e1001403.

Further reading

Anderson IM. Meta-analytical studies on new antidepressants. *Br Med Bull.* 2001;
57: 161–178.

McGirr A, Berlim MT, Bond DJ et al. A systematic review and meta-analysis of randomised, double-blind placebo-controlled trials of ketamine in the rapid treatment of major depressive episodes. *Psychol Med.* 2014; 10: 1–12.

Nelson JC, Baumann P, Delucchi K et al. A systematic review and meta-analysis
of lithium augmentation of tricyclic and second generation antidepressants in
major depression. *J Affect Disord.* 2014; 168: 269–275.

Papakostas G, Fava M, Thase ME. Treatment of SSRI-resistant depression: A meta-
analysis comparing within-versus across-class switches. *Biol Psychiatry.* 2008;
63: 699–704.

Papakostas GI, Thase ME, Fava M et al. Are antidepressant drugs that combine
serotonergic and noradrenergic mechanisms of action more effective than the
selective serotonin reuptake inhibitors in treating major depressive disorder? A
meta-analysis of studies of newer agents. *Biol Psychiatry* 2007; 62: 1217–1227.

Ruhe HG, Huyser J, Swinkels JA et al. Switching antidepressants after a first selective
serotonin reuptake inhibitor in major depressive disorder: A systematic review.
J Clin Psychiatry. 2006; 67: 1836–1855.

Waite J, Easton A (Eds.). *ECT Handbook* (3rd edn.). Royal College of Psychiatrists,
London, 2013.

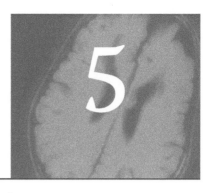

'Mood stabilisers' and other treatments for bipolar disorder

Allan H Young and Sarah C Wooderson

What is a mood stabiliser?

- The term 'mood stabiliser' refers to the ability of a drug to treat one or both poles of bipolar disorder without causing a switch to the other pole (cf. antidepressants which can cause a switch to mania) and historically has tended to be used for drugs used in prophylaxis.
- It has traditionally been applied to lithium and anticonvulsant drugs used to treat bipolar disorder (as well as borderline personality disorder and schizoaffective disorder). It is also starting to be applied to some atypical antipsychotics that have efficacy for both poles or for maintenance treatment of bipolar disorder.
- There are however problems in its use:
  - The evidence for efficacy of drugs is often clearer for one pole than the other.
  - Should it only be applied to drugs that are effective against both poles?
  - Does it refer to acute or maintenance treatment, or both?
- One suggestion is that drugs can be classified as those that treat from above (i.e. mania), called *type A mood stabilisers*; those that treat from below (i.e. depression), called *type B mood stabilisers*; and those that are both type A and type B.
- Some advocate simply referring to a drug's antimanic or antidepressive properties, specifying acute or maintenance treatment and abandoning the term 'mood stabiliser' altogether.

Lithium

History

- Lithium is an alkaline metal element that occurs naturally as the mineral petalite. It is widely used today in swimming pool filters and batteries for mobile phones and computers.
- The Australian psychiatrist John Cade first proposed the use of lithium salts to treat 'psychotic excitement' in 1949, although its sedative and depressant properties had been known since at least the preceding century, and possibly since antiquity.
- Lithium salts were once used extensively as a treatment for gout because lithium urate is particularly soluble and promotes the excretion of urates, reducing their deposition in tissue.
- Lithium chloride was briefly used as a sodium salt substitute before its toxicity was properly appreciated.
- Since the 1960s, lithium has been a first-line maintenance treatment for bipolar disorder.
- Lithium is found to a variable level in drinking water, and higher environmental lithium levels are associated with reduced suicide mortality, consistent with findings in clinical trials.
- Worrisome adverse effects (e.g. renal failure) may be markedly reduced with careful monitoring of lithium and ensuring good compliance is essential.
- As evidence of lithium's efficacy has accumulated, there has been a paradoxical decline in its use; however, increasing evidence, and the NICE (2014) bipolar disorder clinical guideline which promotes lithium's use, may reverse this.

Mechanism of action

Lithium alters the signal induced by multiple neurotransmitter systems, allowing mediation of complex behavioural and physiological responses (see Chapter 1). It is widely believed that these mechanisms account for the efficacy of the drug, although its exact mode of action is unknown.

Cation transport

- Increases the activity of Na^+/K^+ adenosine triphosphatase (ATPase) in patients (but, interestingly, not in healthy controls).
- May displace Ca^{2+} and Mg^{2+} ions at a range of sites relevant to neural function, for example modulation of Ca^{2+}-dependent activities in the CNS, such as neurotransmitter release.

Monoaminergic neurotransmission

- Decreases dopamine (DA) release from the presynaptic neuron
- Increases the synthesis and release of 5-HT
- Increases transmission at 5-HT_{1A} receptors
- Decreases transmission at 5-HT_2 receptors
- Enhances platelet 5-HT uptake
- Increases noradrenaline (NA) uptake into synaptosomes
- May reduce NA turnover overall in humans

Cholinergic neurotransmission

- Increases choline levels.
- Enhances acetylcholinesterase inhibitor toxicity.
- Increases the growth hormone response to cholinergic agonist pyridostigmine.
- These findings suggest that lithium enhances cholinergic activity in the brain. It is conceivable that these cholinomimetic effects may contribute to antimanic actions, while lithium toxicity resembles atropine poisoning.

Effects on second messengers

- Lithium has many interactions with intracellular 'second messenger' systems and can thus modify signal transduction pathways (see Chapter 1):
  - Inhibits Na^+-induced cAMP activity.
  - Inhibits inositol trisphosphate (IP_3) formation.
  - Recent evidence for inhibition of glycogen synthase kinase 3 beta (GSK-3β), involved in energy metabolism and neuronal cell development, may underlie lithium's neuroprotective effects. GSK-3β inhibitors are currently being tested for therapeutic effects in Alzheimer's disease (see Chapter 8), diabetes, cancer and bipolar disorder.

Neuroprotective effects

- Recent evidence that lithium has protective effects on neuronal function and integrity (potentially important because bipolar disorder is associated with structural brain changes):
  - In animal studies, and in isolated human neural cells, lithium increases the expression of neuroprotective proteins.
  - In bipolar patients, lithium appears to increase both grey matter volume and N-acetylaspartate concentrations (a putative marker of neuronal viability).
  - Lithium enhances neurogenesis in rat hippocampus.

- Effects of lithium on both grey and white matter have been suggested as a mechanism by which it reduces suicidal behaviour through effects on executive function.
- Neuroprotective effects may contribute to lithium's long-term benefits in the treatment of mood disorders and suggest potential therapeutic properties in neurodegenerative disorders.

Pharmacokinetics

- Rapidly absorbed in the upper gastrointestinal tract.
- Peak serum levels are achieved within 2–3 h.
- Delayed release preparations attempt to smooth plasma concentration fluctuations.
- Unbound in serum.
- Excreted unchanged by the kidney at a constant rate proportional to the glomerular filtration rate (GFR).
- Steady-state plasma concentration is achieved after 5–7 days.
- Individual lithium preparations have different bioavailability and cannot be substituted dose for dose, so lithium should be prescribed by trade name.

Indications

Acute mania

- In clinical trials, lithium is effective in 60%–80% of acutely ill patients.
- Poorer responses are seen in patients with mixed affective episodes or a rapid cycling pattern.
- Higher levels required than for prophylaxis (see the section titled 'Clinical use of lithium').
- Historically lithium treatment was a first-line strategy for acute mania in the United States (cf. antipsychotic drugs in Europe due to their greater sedation and faster onset of action). A recent network meta-analysis found that most antipsychotics are more effective than lithium and anticonvulsants in treating mania.
- Lithium should be used cautiously with antipsychotics because of alleged risks of neurotoxicity when lithium is combined with high doses of antipsychotic.

Maintenance treatment and relapse prevention

- A recent meta-analysis found that lithium was more effective than placebo in preventing relapse overall, as well as manic and, probably, depressive episodes; against anticonvulsants it was more effective in preventing manic episodes but not overall relapse or depressive episodes.

- Not all patients benefit from lithium. In initial randomised controlled trials, around 80% of patients were reported to benefit. More recent trials, however, suggest poorer results with 70% of patients relapsing and only 30% having good occupational outcome.
- The decision to commence prophylaxis is based on the frequency and severity of episodes. A traditional rule of thumb has been
  - After two illnesses within 2 years
  - After three illnesses in 5 years
  - After one severe illness
- Recent emphasis on the recurrent and progressive nature of bipolar disorder has led to recommending consideration of prophylaxis after a single manic episode
- The decision to commence lithium prophylaxis needs to consider treatment adherence:
  - Abrupt lithium discontinuation leads to rebound mania (and thus more manic episodes than would have occurred had the drug never been started) and depression. A meta-analysis of 19 published studies on lithium discontinuation found that time to recurrence of affective disorder (mostly mania) was within 3 months for 50% of patients after abruptly stopping the drug.
  - As a result, it has been recommended that patients must take the medication for longer than 2 years without discontinuation for benefits to accrue.
  - Gradual discontinuation appears to reduce the risk of rebound mood episodes.
- There is increasing evidence that lithium may help reduce suicidal ideation and prevent completed suicide.
- Lithium is thought to decrease aggression and impulsivity.

Depression treatment and prophylaxis

- Data are limited on the value of lithium as an acute treatment of *bipolar depression*. A recent study found it comparable to quetiapine, which has established efficacy (see Figure 5.1).
- Lithium has good evidence supporting its use as an augmentation strategy for *unipolar depression* non-responsive to antidepressants (see Chapter 4).
- Lithium is also used in the *prophylaxis of recurrent unipolar depressive disorder*; while the strategy is significantly more effective than placebo, the magnitude of effect is small and continuous antidepressant prescription is more effective than lithium.
- Lithium use has been associated with reduced suicidality in unipolar depression as well as in bipolar disorder.

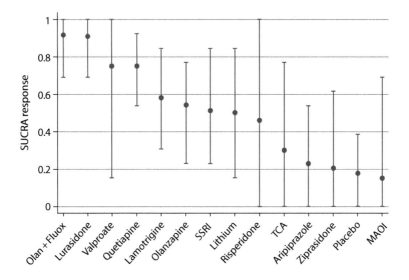

Figure 5.1 Efficacy in rank order for drug treatment of bipolar depression. Surface under the cumulative ranking curve (SUCRA) and 95% confidence intervals are given. SUCRA is a summary statistic for cumulative ranking ranging from 1 (the best treatment with no uncertainty) to 0 (the worst treatment with no uncertainty). (Adapted by permission from Taylor DM et al., *Acta Psychiatr Scand* 2014; 130: 452.)

Other indications

- Prevention of puerperal psychosis
- Prophylaxis in schizoaffective disorder and cyclical schizophrenia
- Adjunct to antipsychotics in schizophrenia
- Reduction in impulsivity
- Reversal of neutropenia

Predicting response to lithium in bipolar disorder (Table 5.1)

Table 5.1 Predictors of response to lithium

Predictors of good response	Predictors of poor response
Positive family history of bipolar disorder	Psychosis
Previous remission with lithium	Substance abuse
Classic euphoric manic episodes	Rapid cycling
Full remission between episodes	More than three episodes
Good adherence	Mixed mania
	Poor compliance

Adverse effects of lithium

Many of the adverse effects are related to serum concentration and may be minimised if levels are kept below 0.8 mmol/L. The adverse effects of lithium are listed in Table 5.2.

Effects on renal function

- Lithium inhibits the action of antidiuretic hormone on the kidney, reducing its ability to concentrate urine causing polyuria (and consequent thirst/polydipsia) and nephrogenic diabetes insipidus (in 10%–40% of patients).
- Polyuria does not predict lasting renal damage and paradoxically may be improved by treatment with the diuretic amiloride. The long-term effects of lithium on renal function are controversial:
  - An early, uncontrolled study found that 21% of patients who had been treated with lithium for more than 15 years had a reduced GFR.

Table 5.2   Adverse effects of lithium

System	Details
Renal (see text)	Thirst, polydipsia, polyuria, impaired renal tubular function, impaired glomerular function (possible)
Gastrointestinal symptoms	Nausea, diarrhoea
Weight gain	
CNS	Mild impairment of attention and memory, tremor
Skin	Precipitates or worsens disorder (e.g. psoriasis, eczema, acne)
Hair loss	
Cardiac	T-wave flattening/inversion on ECG in 30% of patients
Thyroid (see text)	Hypothyroidism and nontoxic goitre (5%–10%); rarely transient hyperthyroidism
Haematological	Leukocytosis
Teratogenicity	Cardiac malformations including Ebstein's anomaly

Note: Avoid a low-sodium diet as this can lead to excessively high lithium levels. Use caution when driving or operating machinery and limit alcoholic beverages.

- Controlled studies have demonstrated few differences between treated and untreated patients with respect to renal pathology. Nevertheless, duration of lithium treatment has been associated with a lower GFR, and about half of patients on lithium for longer than 20 years have a GFR < 60 mL/min/1.73 m², although progression of impairment appears independent of whether lithium is stopped.
- The risk of kidney disease may also relate to intermittently elevated lithium levels, further emphasising the importance of consistent adherence to treatment.
- Given that chronic kidney disease is common, management of lithium treatment in this situation is frequently faced. The decision about whether to continue treatment needs to be based on clinical need and risk, in conjunction with the patient and a renal physician if necessary.

Effects on thyroid function

- Lithium is concentrated in thyroid tissue and inhibits the uptake of iodine into follicular cells, alters the structure of thyroglobulin by interfering with the production of iodothyronines and inhibits the secretion of thyroid hormone and the conversion of thyroxine to active triiodothyronine (T3). Lithium also exacerbates pre-existing thyroid autoimmunity by stimulating immunoglobulin secretion by lymphocytes.
- Lithium treatment is associated with significantly elevated thyroid-stimulating hormone (TSH) concentrations, with a sixfold greater risk of hypothyroidism in lithium-treated compared with control subjects, and can cause goitre. Risk factors include female sex, family history of hypothyroidism, pre-existing elevated TSH, antithyroid antibodies and iodine deficiency.
- Treatment is usually thyroid replacement therapy if lithium treatment remains clinically indicated. Stopping lithium does not necessary lead to normalisation of thyroid function, especially if antithyroid antibodies are present.
- Hyperthyroidism rarely occurs.

Lithium toxicity

- Lithium has a narrow therapeutic index. Signs of toxicity usually appear at serum concentrations > 1.3 mmol/L, although they can occur within the 'therapeutic range' in some individuals:
  - Early features include an exacerbation of existing side effects, including tremor, nausea, vomiting and diarrhoea.

- As toxicity develops, further CNS signs and symptoms occur including disorientation, dysarthria, convulsions and coma.
- Death occurs from cardiac effects or pulmonary complications.
- The investigation of choice in suspected neurotoxicity, which can occur with lithium levels in the therapeutic range, is an EEG to demonstrate characteristic diffuse slowing of cortical activity.
- Management of possible lithium toxicity:
  - Perform an urgent lithium level, renal function and electrolyte tests, and withhold the next lithium dose until result is known. Depending on the cause, early stages are likely to respond to stopping drug and adequate hydration.
  - More severe toxicity is a potentially life-threatening medical emergency requiring admission for rehydration and possibly administration of anticonvulsants.
  - Haemodialysis may be necessary (serum concentration > 3.0 mmol/L, coma supervenes or no response to supportive measures over 24 h).

Drug interactions with lithium

See Table 5.3.

Clinical use of lithium

Safe and effective use of lithium use requires expertise, an informed partnership with the patient and shared care between a psychiatrist and general practitioner. For detailed guidance, consult NICE (2014) and BAP (2009) bipolar disorder treatment guidelines. Important aspects will be highlighted here.

Key points

- Discuss with the patient the need for prolonged treatment (at least 2 years) because of the danger of rebound mania following discontinuation.

Table 5.3 Drug interactions with lithium

Increased lithium levels	CNS toxicity
Diuretics	Antidepressants
Non-steroidal anti-inflammatory drugs	Antipsychotics
Angiotensin-converting enzyme inhibitors	Antihypertensives
	General anaesthetics?

- Education about lithium includes
  - Avoiding suddenly stopping lithium unless for safety reasons
  - Seeking medical help for situations that could increase lithium concentrations; these include fluid loss (dehydration, diarrhoea, vomiting) and before starting non-steroidal anti-inflammatory drugs
  - Seeking advice for intended or actual pregnancy
- Baseline investigations including renal function (serum creatinine/creatinine clearance/estimated GFR) electrolytes, thyroid function, ECG (if cardiac concerns), weight/BMI, pregnancy test if indicated.
- Single daily dosing to achieve therapeutic serum lithium concentration (usually 0.5–0.8 mmol/L for maintenance, but up to 1.0 mmol/L if necessary); higher levels are usually needed for treatment of mania (0.8–1.2 mmol/L, but caution above 1.0 mmol/L).
- Monitoring:
  - Serum lithium concentrations weekly until stable and then 3–6 monthly depending on clinical indications
  - Renal function, electrolytes, thyroid function 3–6 monthly and other baseline assessments as indicated
  - Mood symptoms (consider mood diary) and potential lithium toxicity (paraesthesia, ataxia, tremor and cognitive impairment) at each visit
  - More frequent monitoring if necessary, for example impaired renal function, with a rate of deterioration assessed
- If it becomes necessary to discontinue lithium, this should be slowly done in an effort to reduce the likelihood of rebound episodes of illness or worsening suicidality.

Anticonvulsants

Background

- The use of anticonvulsants has increased in treating bipolar disorder. It has been suggested that similar mechanisms underlie mood stabilisation and seizure control in epilepsy:
  - ECT, which is also a potent anticonvulsant, has strong antidepressive and antimanic actions.
  - There has been speculation that epilepsy and severe affective disorder share some common pathophysiology with a 'kindling'-like acceleration of mood episodes occurring in the natural history of affective disorders, as found with seizures in animals. Most anticonvulsant drugs inhibit the electrically induced kindling of seizure activity in animals.
  - However, not all anticonvulsants are effective mood stabilisers.

- The mode of action of mood-stabilising anticonvulsants is uncertain. A possible common action is to enhance the actions of GABA and thus strengthen inhibitory circuits in the CNS. Effects may also be mediated through actions on membrane excitability or DA neurotransmission.
- The antisuicide effect seen with lithium does not appear to apply to anticonvulsants.

Sodium valproate

- Available in different formulations. Valproate semisodium (called divalproex sodium in the United States) is a mixture of sodium valproate and valproic acid licenced for the treatment of acute mania.
- It is the most frequently prescribed 'mood stabiliser' in the United States and has increasingly been used in Europe.
- A network meta-analysis found that it is less effective than antipsychotics in treating acute mania; evidence in treating bipolar depression is limited (see Figure 5.1) and in maintenance treatment, it appears similar to lithium but may be a little less effective in preventing manic relapse.
- It is no longer restricted to patients who have failed to respond to, or are intolerant of, lithium, and use as first-line monotherapy has increased over the last two decades. However, it has now probably been overtaken by newer (atypical) antipsychotics.

Mode of action

Its mode of action is unclear, but it has a number of effects that may contribute to its therapeutic effects:

- Enhancement of GABAergic function
- Inhibition of GABA-transaminase
- Increase in GABA binding in some brain structures, most notably the hippocampus
- Like lithium, inhibition of protein kinase C
- Reduction in the action of NA at α_2-adrenoceptors
- Antagonism of the functional effects of DA via effects on GABAergic interneurons
- Blockade of voltage-dependent Na^+ channels

Indications

- Antimanic agent (appears most effective in non-psychotic patients).
- Treatment-refractory mania in combination with atypical anti psychotics.
- Rapid cycling bipolar disorder.

- Maintenance treatment of bipolar disorder.
- In epilepsy, valproate is used to treat primary generalised seizures, generalised absences and myoclonic seizures.

Adverse effects

See Table 5.4.

Valproate use in practice

- Valproate is contraindicated in girls and young women of childbearing potential because of the high risk of adverse effects (particularly cognitive) on the foetus (see Use of anticonvulsants in pregancy and laction section and Chapter 11).
- *Monitoring*:
  - Weight.
  - Liver function tests (LFTs) at baseline and in the first 6 months of treatment (clinical vigilance more important).
  - Full blood count (FBC) and clotting indices if clinical indication and before surgery.
  - Pregnancy test if pregnancy possible.
  - It is unclear if serum concentrations are a useful guide to dose but may be helpful in cases of poor response/adherence.
- There is evidence for some dose–response effects in the treatment of mania and loading doses can be considered to speed response in severe illness.
- Valproate semisodium and other valproate preparations do not have the same dose equivalence (higher bioavailability with valproate semisodium); compelling evidence for significantly greater tolerability of valproate semisodium over sodium valproate is lacking.

Table 5.4   Adverse effects of valproate

System	Details
CNS	Tremor, concentration, confusion, headaches
Liver	Hepatotoxicity
Gastrointestinal	Nausea, vomiting, diarrhoea
Blood dyscrasias	
Weight gain	
Lethargy	
Alopecia	
Reproductive	Possibly polycystic ovaries and infertility in women
Teratogenic effects	Heart, neural tube, lip and palate
Effects on children exposed in pregnancy	Cognitive impairment

Carbamazepine

Carbamazepine is licenced in the United Kingdom for the prophylaxis of bipolar disorder unresponsive to lithium and in the United States for mania and mixed episodes.

Mode of action

- The mechanism of the therapeutic effect of carbamazepine is unknown. Although a tricyclic structure like imipramine, it lacks acute monoamine effects.
- Acute effects include stabilisation of inactivated voltage-gated Na^+ channels, making neurons less excitable; potentiation of peripheral benzodiazepine (BDZ)-, α_2- and $GABA_B$-receptor functions; increase in striatal ACh transmission; and decrease in adenylate cyclase activity.
- Chronic administration increases tryptophan availability and substance P and adenosine-A_1 receptor sensitivity.

Indications

- The evidence base for the efficacy of carbamazepine in treating bipolar disorder is limited, with evidence for antimanic efficacy similar to lithium and possible efficacy in bipolar depression. It appears to have inferior efficacy compared to lithium in preventing relapse.
- Limited evidence suggests that carbamazepine may be effective in treatment-resistant mania and treatment-resistant schizophrenia.
- Its use now tends to be as an adjunct to other agents in the prophylaxis of poorly controlled bipolar affective disorder and historically has been considered to have value in rapid cycling bipolar disorder.
- Although the drug has been used in recurrent unipolar depression and treatment-resistant depressive disorder, there is little convincing evidence to support this.
- In epilepsy, carbamazepine is used for partial or generalised tonic–clonic seizures and for trigeminal neuralgia.

Adverse effects (Table 5.5)

- Although traditionally regarded by some psychiatrists as a 'safer' alternative to lithium, carbamazepine has a range of potentially serious side effects (Table 5.5) and patient tolerance is poor. Many of the autoimmune effects are thought to be related to the metabolite carbamazepine-10,11-epoxide.
- Weight gain appears less of a problem than with lithium or valproate.

Table 5.5   Adverse effects of carbamazepine

System	Details
CNS	Headache, dizziness, drowsiness, diplopia
Liver	Elevation of hepatic enzymes, hepatitis, cholestatic jaundice
Gastrointestinal	Nausea, vomiting
Blood dyscrasias	
Skin rashes	Includes serious reactions including toxic epidermal necrolysis and Stevens–Johnson syndrome
Teratogenic effects	Possibly related to folate deficiency, including spina bifida

Interactions

Carbamazepine has important pharmacokinetic interactions:

- It induces the metabolism of
  - Anticoagulants
  - Psychotropic drugs including antidepressants, antipsychotics, sodium valproate and BDZs
  - Oral contraceptives (leading to contraceptive failure)
  - Steroids
- Drugs increasing carbamazepine concentrations include valproic acid, Ca^{2+} channel blockers, cimetidine, erythromycin and grapefruit juice.
- Drugs decreasing carbamazepine concentrations include phenytoin and phenobarbital.
- Carbamazepine is contraindicated in patients receiving clozapine (enhances risk of blood dyscrasia).

Carbamazepine use in practice

- Extended release formulations appear better tolerated than immediate release ones, with fewer autonomic and GI adverse events.
- There is no good evidence for a relationship between serum carbamazepine concentrations and efficacy. Most studies have used 600 mg daily or above.
- Carbamazepine should be stopped at the first sign of rash unless clearly not drug-related. Serious dermatological reactions (e.g. Stevens–Johnson syndrome [SJS]) tend to occur in the first few months of treatment, and certain populations are strongly associated with particular human leucocyte antigen (HLA) types. Screening for HLA-B*1502 is recommended for those with Chinese and other Asian ancestry,

with avoidance of carbamazepine if positive. HLA-A*3101 raises the risk in those with European and Japanese ancestry but the value of screening is uncertain (see Further reading for UK MHRA and US FDA recommendations).

- Clinical advice about, and monitoring for, blood, hepatic and skin disorders is recommended but the practical benefit of routine blood monitoring (FBC and LFTs) is not established.

Oxcarbazepine

- Related to carbamazepine and has a common active metabolite, 10,11-dihydroxycarbamazepine.
- Compared with carbamazepine,
    - It is not metabolised to carbamazepine-10,11-epoxide and lacks the same propensity to cause autoimmune reactions and rashes.
    - It causes less hepatic enzyme induction and so has fewer drug–drug interactions.
- There is a small controlled trial suggesting antimanic efficacy but only limited evidence in prophylaxis, making its place in the treatment of bipolar disorder unclear.
- Similar indications to carbamazepine in epilepsy.

Lamotrigine

- Licenced in the United States and EU for prevention of depressive relapse in bipolar disorder.
- Inhibits voltage-sensitive Na^+ channels, leading to stabilisation of neuronal membranes, and also blocks Ca^{2+} channels and is a weak $5-HT_3$ antagonist.
- Has modest antidepressant activity (see Figure 5.1) but lacks acute antimanic effects. In bipolar prophylaxis, lamotrigine prevents depressive relapse and possibly manic relapse but is less effective than lithium for the latter.
- Its use is mainly as an adjunctive treatment.
- Side effects include rash (5%–10%), dizziness and loss of balance, blurred vision, insomnia, GI symptoms.
- Serious dermatological reactions, including SJS, can occur, especially early in treatment, in the young, and with rapid increases in dose. Aseptic meningitis has also been described so that rash and fever need urgent medical attention.
- Slow titration and avoidance of rapid reinstatement after discontinuation lower the risk of dermatological reactions. Its dose should be halved when used with valproate which inhibits its metabolism.

Other anticonvulsants

Although other anticonvulsants have been investigated as treatments for bipolar disorder, none have unequivocal evidence for efficacy or an established place in treatment.

Phenytoin

- Used in the treatment of epilepsy, trigeminal neuralgia and as a cardiac arrhythmic.
- Principal action is to block voltage-gated Na^+ channels and is a class 1b antiarrhythmic.
- One research group has found suggestive evidence for antimanic and prophylactic effects in bipolar disorder.
- It is not indicated for treatment of bipolar disorder due to its narrow therapeutic range, adverse effects, teratogenicity and induction of CYP450 enzymes.

Topiramate

- Used for the treatment of epilepsy, Lennox–Gastaut syndrome and migraine.
- Actions include blockade of voltage-gated Na^+ channels, high-voltage-activated Ca^{2+} channels, $GABA_A$ receptors, AMPA/kainate glutamate receptors and carbonic anhydrase isoenzymes.
- In spite of early optimism, it has not proved effective in the treatment of bipolar disorder.
- Side effects include dizziness, weight loss, paraesthesia, sedation, GI symptoms and cognitive impairment.
- It is licenced in the United States for weight loss and has been used for the treatment of drug-induced weight gain in psychiatric disorders, although not recommended for this.

Tiagabine

- An anticonvulsant used as adjunctive treatment for partial seizures, which reduces the reuptake of GABA into neuronal and glial cells. It has also been used as an off-label adjunctive treatment for anxiety disorders.
- Elevated brain levels of GABA have been reported in patients with euthymic bipolar disorder using nuclear magnetic spectroscopy, and therefore in theory this may be reversed by tiagabine.
- Small early open studies have provided conflicting evidence of benefit in bipolar disorder, and it has not been tested in controlled trials.

Levetiracetam

▦ Used as monotherapy for partial seizures and adjunctive therapy for partial and general seizures. Its mechanism of action is unknown but it binds to a synaptic vesicle glycoprotein and inhibits presynaptic Ca^{2+} channels.

▦ There is equivocal open evidence in mania. Small randomised trials have not demonstrated adjunctive benefit for mania or bipolar depression.

Zonisamide

▦ Used as adjunctive therapy for partial and generalised seizures and Lennox–Gastaut syndrome.

▦ Blocks Na^+ and Ca^{2+} channels, is a weak carbonic anhydrase inhibitor and modulates GABAergic and glutamatergic neurotransmission.

▦ Open studies have suggested possible efficacy in mania and bipolar depression, but an RCT of adjunctive zonisamide in mania failed to demonstrate efficacy.

▦ It causes weight loss when used in adjunctive therapy, and a placebo-controlled RCT found that it prevented olanzapine-induced weight gain, but at the cost of cognitive impairment.

Antipsychotics (see Chapter 3)

▦ Typical and atypical antipsychotics are widely used in bipolar disorder and antimanic efficacy appears to be a class effect (including in relapse prevention). Traditionally, they have been first-line agents for treating mania in Europe, whereas lithium, anticonvulsants and BDZs have been preferred in the United States.

▦ A network meta-analysis found that antipsychotics are in general more effective than lithium and mood stabilisers in the treatment of mania, with haloperidol showing the greatest effect size.

▦ Antipsychotics differ in their antidepressant effects, but some newer, atypical, drugs show unequivocal efficacy (see Figure 5.1).

▦ Side effects associated with older, typical, antipsychotics, and concern that they may cause depression, have led to a decline in their use in prophylaxis.

▦ Recent RCT evidence for atypical antipsychotics:
  - Has confirmed acute antimanic effects for all that have been studied (no trials with lurasidone, amisulpride and zotepine).
  - A network meta-analysis of treatment in bipolar depression found that olanzapine combined with fluoxetine (licenced in the United States), quetiapine and lurasidone were most effective with

olanzapine and risperidone appearing less effective. Aripiprazole and ziprasidone were ineffective (Figure 5.1).
- Quetiapine is effective in preventing manic and depressive relapse, and olanzapine is effective in preventing manic more than depressive relapse.

Antidepressants (see Chapter 4)

- The use of antidepressants in bipolar disorder has generally been discouraged because of their ability to switch patients into mania, although this is less likely with SSRIs than drugs with NA activity (SNRIs, TCAs and monoamine oxidase inhibitors [MAOIs]), or in the presence of an antimanic agent.
- Good evidence for benefit in the acute treatment of bipolar depression already optimally treated with a mood stabiliser, or for prophylaxis of depressive relapse, is lacking.
- A recent network meta-analysis supports the efficacy of SSRIs in bipolar depression, but not TCAs or MAOIs (Figure 5.1). Other meta-analyses have been negative.
- In practice, antidepressants
  - Are used relatively frequently because of the difficulty in treating bipolar depression
  - Should not be used in bipolar disorder without concomitant use of an antimanic agent
  - Are not recommended for routine long-term use in bipolar disorder, although clinically they may be beneficial for some patients

Benzodiazepines (see Chapter 6)

- BDZs are useful in adjunctive treatment of manic excitement and agitation, but there is no evidence they treat the underlying mood disorder.
- They are used in the United States in combination with lithium or valproate in preference to antipsychotics for the treatment of less severe acute mania.

Use of mood stabilisers in pregnancy and lactation (see also Chapter 11)

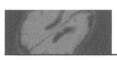

- Specialist preconception advice is advised for women with bipolar disorder and pregnancy should be jointly management by psychiatric and obstetric services, with careful monitoring of foetal development.

- There is a high risk of bipolar relapse, especially depressive, during pregnancy; one study found about a quarter relapsed during pregnancy and a half in the postpartum period. Risk is increased if mood stabilisers are stopped.
- Lithium and anticonvulsants are associated with an increased risk of teratogenicity. This is greatest with valproate, which also causes neurodevelopmental delay in 30%–40% of children exposed prenatally.
- Valproate is contraindicated in women of childbearing age and, if used, effective contraception is needed. It is absolutely contraindicated in pregnancy.
- Lithium and other anticonvulsants are contraindicated in the first trimester; continuation needs to be carefully balanced against the risk of stopping the drug.
- Antipsychotics are the antimanic treatment of choice during pregnancy. Consider psychological treatment for treating depression, otherwise a drug other than lithium or an anticonvulsant.
- Lithium should be stopped during labour. After delivery reinstate, or start, effective drug treatment to prevent relapse.
- Lithium and carbamazepine are contraindicated in breast feeding (see Chapter 11).

Treatment issues

- Treatment of bipolar disorder is complex due to the often chaotic nature of the illness, different phases and presentations and continuing symptoms and impaired functioning between major relapses. The treatment of bipolar II disorder and bipolar spectrum disorders are particularly under-researched.
- Mania is the most disruptive phase, but nearly always responds well to treatment. There are fewer effective evidence-based treatments for depression which is less responsive to treatment. The high risk of recurrence means that prophylactic treatment is nearly always required, but efficacy is limited, especially in those with frequent relapse or rapid cycling.
- Only a minority of patients can be maintained on a single agent. There is limited evidence about the most effective way to combine different agents and the place of antidepressants in treatment. Greater efficacy for combination over monotherapy has been found for
  - Antipsychotic + lithium/mood stabiliser > monotherapy for mania
  - Antipsychotic + lithium/mood stabiliser > lithium/mood stabiliser in preventing manic relapse
  - Quetiapine + lithium/mood stabiliser > lithium/mood stabiliser in preventing manic and depressive relapse
  - Lithium + valproate > valproate in preventing any relapse

- Adjunctive psychological treatment reduces relapse with the strongest evidence for group psychoeducation and family-focused therapy.
- If discontinuing mood stabilisers they should be stopped gradually, even if an individual has started to take another antimanic drug.

Acknowledgement

This is an update and revision of the third edition chapter which was contributed to by Ian C Reid.

Bibliography

Guidelines

Goodwin GM for the Consensus Group of the British Association for Psychopharmacology. Evidence-based guidelines for treating bipolar disorder (revised 2nd edn.) – Recommendations from the British Association for Psychopharmacology. *J Psychopharmacol.* 2009; 23: 346–388. http://www.bap.org.uk/pdfs/Bipolar_guidelines.pdf.

National Institute for Health and Care Excellence. Bipolar disorder: The assessment and management of bipolar disorder in adults, children and young people in primary and secondary care. *NICE Clinical Guideline 185.* 2014; http://www.nice.org.uk/guidance/cg185.

Yatham LN, Kennedy SH, Parikh SV et al. Canadian Network for Mood and Anxiety Treatments (CANMAT) and International Society for Bipolar Disorders (ISBD) collaborative update of CANMAT guidelines for the management of patients with bipolar disorder: Update 2013. *Bipolar Disord.* 2013; 15: 1–44.

Key references

Achieving success in the management of bipolar disorder: Is lithium enough? A series of articles on lithium and alternatives in treating bipolar disorder. *J Clin Psychiatry.* 2003; 64(Suppl. 5).

Anderson IM, Haddad PM, Scott J. Bipolar disorder. *BMJ.* 2012; 345: e8508.

Cipriani A, Hawton K, Stockton S, Geddes, JR. Lithium in the prevention of suicide in mood disorders: Updated systematic review and meta-analysis. *BMJ.* 2013; 346: f3646.

Cipriani A, Barbui C, Salanti G et al. Comparative efficacy and acceptability of antimanic drugs in acute mania: A multiple-treatments meta-analysis. *Lancet.* 2011; 378(9799): 1306–1315.

Gijsman HJ, Geddes JR, Rendell JM et al. Antidepressants for bipolar depression: A systematic review of randomized, controlled trials. *Am J Psychiatry.* 2004; 161: 1537–1547.

Kessing LV, Vradi E, Andersen PK. Starting lithium prophylaxis early v. late in bipolar disorder. *Br J Psychiatry.* 2014; 205: 214–220.

Kohler S, Gaus S, Bschor T. The challenge of treatment in bipolar depression: Evidence from clinical guidelines, treatment recommendations and complex treatment situations. *Pharmacopsychiatry.* 2014; 47: 53–59.

Nelson JC, Baumann P, Delucchi K et al. A systematic review and meta-analysis of lithium augmentation of tricyclic and second generation antidepressants in major depression. *J Affect Disord.* 2014; 168: 269–275.

Pacchiarotti I, Bond DJ, Baldessarini RJ et al. The International Society for Bipolar Disorders (ISBD) task force report on antidepressant use in bipolar disorders. *Am J Psychiatry.* 2013; 170: 1249–1262.

Severus E, Taylor MJ, Sauer C et al. Lithium for prevention of mood episodes in bipolar disorders: Systematic review and meta-analysis. *Int J Bipolar Disord.* 2014; 2: 15.

Taylor DM, Cornelius V, Smith L, Youn AH. Comparative efficacy and acceptability of drug treatments for bipolar depression: A multiple-treatments meta-analysis. *Acta Psychiatr Scand.* 2014; 130: 452–469.

Young AH and Hammond JM. Lithium in mood disorders: Increasing evidence base, declining use? *Br J Psychiatry.* 2007; 191: 474–476.

Further reading

Aiff H, Attman PO, Aurell M et al. The impact of modern treatment principles may have eliminated lithium-induced renal failure. *J Psychopharmacol.* 2014; 28: 151–154.

Benedetti F, Poletti S, Radaelli D et al. Lithium and GSK-3β promoter gene variants influence cortical gray matter volumes in bipolar disorder. *Psychopharmacology.* 2015; 232: 1325–1336.

Bond K, Anderson IM. Psychoeducation for relapse prevention in bipolar disorder: A systematic review of efficacy in randomized controlled trials. *Bipolar Disord.* 2015; 17: 349–362.

Cochrane Reviews: Bipolar Disorder. The Cochrane Library has a number of systematic reviews and meta-analyses of individual drugs. http://www.thecochranelibrary.com/details/browseReviews/576821/Bipolar-disorder.html.

Diav-Citrin O, Shechtman S, Tahover E et al. Pregnancy outcome following in utero exposure to lithium: A prospective, comparative, observational study. *Am J Psychiatry.* 2014; 171: 785–794.

Gitlin M. Treatment-resistant bipolar disorder. *Mol Psychiatry.* 2006; 11: 227–240.

Goodwin GM. Recurrence of mania after lithium withdrawal: Implications for the use of lithium in the treatment of bipolar affective disorder. *Br J Psychiatry.* 1994; 164: 149–152.

Gray JD, McEwen BS. Lithium's role in neural plasticity and its implications for mood disorders. *Acta Psychiatr Scand.* 2013; 128: 347–361.

Medicines and Healthcare Products Regulatory Agency. Drug Safety Update: Carbamazepine, oxcarbazepine and eslicarbazepine: Potential risk of serious skin reactions. 2012; https://www.gov.uk/drug-safety-update/carbamazepine-oxcarbazepine-and-eslicarbazepine-potential-risk-of-serious-skin-reactions.

US Food and Drug Administration. Information for Healthcare Professionals: Dangerous or Even Fatal Skin Reactions - Carbamazepine (marketed as Carbatrol, Equetro, Tegretol, and generics). 2013; http://www.fda.gov/Drugs/DrugSafety/PostmarketDrugSafetyInformationforPatientsandProviders/ucm124718.htm.

Yildiz A, Ruiz P, Nemeroff C (Eds.). *The Bipolar Book: History, Neurobiology, and Treatment.* Oxford, UK: Oxford University Press, 2015.

Yonkers KA, Wisner KL, Stowe Z et al. Management of bipolar disorder during pregnancy and the postpartum period. *Am J Psychiatry.* 2004; 161: 608–620.

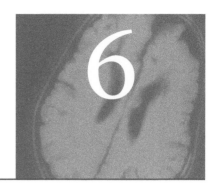

Anxiolytic and hypnotic drugs

6

David S Baldwin and Nupur Tiwari

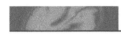 ## Brief history

- *Pre-benzodiazepine era*
  - Bromides, chloral and paraldehyde were introduced in the nineteenth century.
  - Barbiturates, meprobamate and related compounds became available early in the twentieth century, but were found to have a low therapeutic index: In the United Kingdom between 1959 and 1974, there were 27,000 deaths associated with barbiturates, and 225 million prescriptions.
  - Nevertheless, barbiturates were the predominant prescribed anxiolytics until the introduction of benzodiazepines (BDZs).
- *Benzodiazepine era*
  - Chlordiazepoxide ('Librium') became available in 1960, soon followed (1963) by diazepam ('Valium'). There was a rapid growth in clinical use, peaking in about 1979.
  - BDZ found to have a higher therapeutic index than barbiturates, but awareness of tolerance, dependence and withdrawal problems at usual therapeutic doses in a proportion of patients (first fully recognised in the early 1980s) led to reduced prescribing and recommendations that prescriptions should be avoided or only short term.
- *Post-benzodiazepine era*
  - Buspirone, a 5-HT$_{1A}$ partial agonist, became available in the mid-1980s.
  - Trials with SSRIs in anxiety disorders started shortly after. SSRIs are now recommended first-line pharmacological treatments for anxiety disorders.
  - SNRIs were evaluated later, and both venlafaxine and duloxetine are licensed for the treatment of generalised anxiety disorder (GAD).
  - Pregabalin, a non-BDZ anxiolytic (also with anticonvulsant and analgesic properties), is licensed for treatment of GAD in many countries.

 Neurobiology of anxiety

Brain aversion system

Different anxiety, and anxiety-related, disorders (Table 6.1) are believed to reflect, at least in part, altered function in different components/combinations of components of the brain aversion system. For simplicity, obsessive–compulsive disorder (OCD) and post-traumatic stress disorder (PTSD) are included under anxiety disorders in this chapter, although they are considered as distinct disorders by many.

Table 6.1 Main anxiety and anxiety-related disorders

Generalised anxiety disorder
Persistent excessive and inappropriate worrying, not restricted to particular circumstances. Comorbidity with depression and other anxiety disorders is common.

Panic disorder (with or without agoraphobia)
Recurrent unexpected panic attacks (surges of severe anxiety) with variable anticipatory anxiety between attacks. Agoraphobia (fear and avoidance of situations where escape, or getting help, is difficult) develops in about two-thirds of patients.

Social phobia (social anxiety disorder)
Marked, persistent and unreasonable fear of being observed or evaluated negatively by others in social situations.

Specific phobia (simple phobia and isolated phobia)
Excessive or unreasonable fear of (and restricted to) single people, animals, objects or situations.

Separation anxiety disorder
Excessive or persistent anxiety concerning separation from, or worry about, those to whom an individual is attached.

Post-traumatic stress disorder
A history of exposure to trauma leading to subsequent intrusive and distressing re-experiencing of the event, avoidance, negative thoughts and mood and hyperarousal.

Obsessive–compulsive disorder
Recurrent distressing and time-consuming obsessive ruminations, images or impulses and/or recurrent physical or mental rituals and touching.

Illness anxiety disorder
Excessive or disproportionate preoccupations, alarms and behaviours related to having, or acquiring, a serious illness.

- *Periaqueductal grey (PAG)*
  - Brainstem area
  - Linked to stereotyped, 'hard-wired' responses of fight or flight
  - Panic attacks likely to be linked to activation of PAG – spontaneous panics may originate at this level
- *Medial hypothalamus*
  - Autonomic and endocrine components of anxiety response
- *Amygdala*
  - Important role in classical conditioning and coordinating/integrating fear responses
  - Response to cues and close threat (e.g. startle reactions) with inputs from thalamus
  - Contains chemosensors sensitive to changes in blood pH
- *Septohippocampal system*
  - Role in context of anxiety and inhibition of behaviour
  - Likely role in avoidance and anticipatory anxiety
- *Temporal and prefrontal cortex*
  - Higher-order processing, including of social situations
  - Likely role in anticipatory and socially induced anxiety

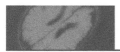 **Neurotransmitter systems** (see also Chapter 1)

Noradrenaline/norepinephrine (NA)

- There are three major 'families' of adrenoceptors (α_1, α_2 and β): All are members of the G-protein-coupled receptor 'superfamily'.
- NA acts mainly through α-adrenoceptors and adrenaline through β-adrenoceptors.
- NA is critical in the fast response to stress and seems to remain hyper-reactive in chronic anxiety states.
- Physiological symptoms of anxiety in humans are consistent with features of adrenergic 'overactivity'.
- α-Adrenoceptor antagonists reduce physiological symptoms of anxiety.
- Yohimbine (α_2 antagonist) infusion increases NA release and causes panic in panic disorder patients but has little effect in non-anxious subjects.
- Clonidine (α_2 agonist) infusion causes decreased NA release and may decrease anxiety in some situations.

Serotonin (5-HT)

- 5-HT_{1A} partial agonists (e.g. buspirone) decrease anxiety in GAD but are not effective in panic disorder.

▦ Some 5-HT$_2$ agonists (e.g. *m*-chlorophenylpiperazine, a metabolite of trazodone and nefazodone) are anxiogenic.

▦ SSRIs are effective in treating all anxiety disorders – GAD, panic disorder, social anxiety disorder, simple (specific) phobia – and also PTSD and OCD.

▦ Anxiety symptoms are sometimes worsened in the initial phase of pharmacological treatment with SSRIs.

▦ 5-HT has a complex role in anxiety
   – In animal models, the effect of 5-HT depends on the model and anxiety situation being examined.
   – 5-HT acts at different levels of the brain aversion system, inhibiting brainstem hard-wired panic system but increasing anxiety in temporal lobe structures involved in conditioned/generalised anxiety.

▦ There is 'crosstalk' between neurotransmitters, for example one theory: ↑5-HT release → ↑frontal cortex stimulation → ↓activity of GABA projection to locus coeruleus (LC) → ↑LC firing.

GABA

▦ GABA is the most widely distributed inhibitory neuro transmitter.

▦ GABA$_A$ receptors have wide distribution in the central nervous system (CNS) and are involved in most brain functions, including the brain aversion system.

▦ BDZs (which enhance GABA$_A$ function) are effective in treatment of most anxiety disorders.

▦ Pentylenetetrazol (inhibitor of GABA$_A$–BDZ receptor) causes extreme anxiety symptoms and seizures.

▦ Flumazenil (BDZ inhibitor) may cause panic in panic patients but not in non-anxious subjects (possibly indicates an abnormality of BDZ receptor sensitivity in panic disorder).

▦ BDZ receptor number (measured by PET studies of flumazenil binding) is reduced by 20% in panic disorder.

▦ Mice genetically altered to have only 50% of α_2-subunits (linked to BDZ-binding site) in GABA$_A$–BDZ receptors (*receptor 'knockout'*) have behavioural equivalent of anxiety.

▦ Effect of BDZs may involve acting on receptors on monoamine neurons, for example brainstem and LC leading to reduced NA and 5-HT neuronal firing.

Glutamate

▦ The predominant excitatory neurotransmitter within the CNS

▦ Receptors are either ionotropic (with sensitivity for NMDA, AMPA or kainic acid) or metabotropic (mGluRs) (with effects being mediated by second messenger systems)

- A range of ligands at ionotropic and metabotropic receptors can mediate 'anxiolytic' (and sometimes 'anxiogenic') effects in animal models: NMDA and AMPA receptor antagonists are generally anxiolytic; antagonists at mGluR1 and mGluR5 have been found to exert anxiolytic effects
- The NMDA receptor partial agonist D-cycloserine facilitates extinction of fear and has been found (though inconsistently) to enhance the effectiveness of cognitive behaviour therapy for phobic anxiety disorders

Cholecystokinin

- Infusion of cholecystokinin tetrapeptide (CCK4) and pentagastrin (agonists at CCKB receptors) induces panic in humans.
- CCKB receptor antagonists are anxiolytic in some animal models, but have not been effective in clinical trials, possibly because of poor CNS penetration.

Carbon dioxide (CO_2) sensitivity

- Increased sensitivity to inhaled 35% CO_2 in panic disorder leads to panic anxiety.
- Inhalation of 7.5% CO_2 provides a robust model of generalised anxiety.
- Lactate infusion (possibly by altering acid–base balance) provokes panic in anxious patients.
- These findings are consistent with possible alterations of brainstem sensitivity to CO_2.

Immunological disturbances

- Acute stress can engender inflammatory reactions, with increased levels of pro-inflammatory cytokines.
- Chronic anxiety is associated with deleterious effects on cellular and humoral immune responses.
- Trait anxiety in healthy populations is associated with increased levels of markers of inflammation and coagulation such as tumour necrosis factor-α, interleukin-6 and C-reactive protein.

Pharmacology of sleep and wakefulness

- The balance of sleepiness and wakefulness depends on a number of neurotransmitter systems (Table 6.2).
- Activating neurotransmitters include NA, 5-HT, ACh, DA, histamine and orexin.

Table 6.2 Wakefulness- and sleep-promoting systems

Sleep-promoting system
GABAergic – Ventrolateral preoptic nucleus of the hypothalamus
Wakefulness-promoting system
NAergic – Locus coeruleus
Histaminergic – Tuberomammillary nucleus
Orexinergic – Lateral hypothalamus/perifornical area
Cholinergic – Pedunculopontine tegmental nucleus
5-HTergic – Dorsal raphé nucleus
DAergic – Ventral tegmental area
Glutamatergic – Thalamus (intralaminar nuclei)
Sleep and arousal modulators
Melatonin, adenosine and galanin

- Promotion of sleep is influenced by GABA (through $GABA_A$ receptors), adenosine (adenosine-A2 receptors are blocked by caffeine) and melatonin (affects circadian pacemaker in the suprachiasmatic nucleus).
- Slow-release melatonin is licensed for the short-term treatment of primary insomnia in older adults, and the melatonin receptor agonist, ramelteon, is licensed in the United States for insomnia (particularly with delayed sleep onset).

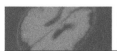 # Drugs used to treat anxiety disorders and insomnia

Benzodiazepines

Pharmacology of Benzodiazepines

See Chapter 1 and Figure 1.13 for a fuller description of GABA receptors. Only selected details are given here.

- $GABA_A$ receptors include binding sites for BDZ, barbiturates and neurosteroids ('$GABA_A$–BDZ complex').
- Endogenous ligands for the BDZ site have been identified, but their function is unknown.
- If GABA is absent or the $GABA_A$ receptor is blocked (e.g. by bicuculline in vitro), BDZs will have no effect, making them relatively safe in overdose (unlike barbiturates, which open the Cl⁻ channel in the absence of GABA, resulting in respiratory depression).

- Newer hypnotic drugs modulate the $GABA_A$–BDZ complex but have some pharmacodynamic differences to BDZ
  - Zolpidem and zaleplon are relatively selective for α_1 subunits.
  - Zopiclone binds to a different site to BDZs and zolpidem.
- Drugs binding at the BDZ site may have inhibitory or stimulatory effects on GABA function (see Chapter 2 for discussion of agonism and inverse agonism)
  - Full agonists (e.g. diazepam) and partial agonists (e.g. clonazepam) at the BDZ receptor act to *enhance* the action of GABA.
  - Full and partial inverse agonists *inhibit* the action of GABA (e.g. ethyl-β-carboline-3-carboxylate), increase anxiety and are pro-convulsant. There are no clinically useful drugs in this category at present.
  - Neutral antagonists occupy BDZ-binding sites and so prevent the action of agonists or inverse agonists (e.g. flumazenil).
- BDZs have little direct effect on autonomic, cardiovascular or respiratory function unless given intravenously.
- BDZs do not induce hepatic enzyme induction.
- Many BDZs undergo Phase I metabolism to produce active metabolites (Table 6.3) which
  - Generally have a longer elimination half-life than the 'parent' compound
  - May lead to prolonged effects if their plasma concentration rises
  - May be largely responsible for 'hangover' effects when using BDZ regularly as a hypnotic
  - May contribute to confusion in susceptible subjects (e.g. the elderly)

Table 6.3 Pharmacokinetic parameters for some benzodiazepines and similar compounds

Drug	Absorption	Half-life (parent drug) (h)	Metabolic phases	Half-life (active metabolite)	Clinical use
Diazepam	Rapid	20–100	I + II	30–90 h	Anxiolytic
Alprazolam	Intermediate	5–15	I + II	Very low concentration	Antipanic
Lorazepam	Intermediate	10–20	II only	None	Anxiolytic
Nitrazepam	Intermediate	24	I + II	30–90 h	Hypnotic
Flurazepam	Rapid	2	I + II	30–100 h	Hypnotic
Temazepam	Slow	10	II only	None	Hypnotic
Zolpidem	Rapid	2	II only	None	Hypnotic
Zopiclone	Rapid	4	I + II	3–6 h	Hypnotic
Zaleplon	Rapid	1	II only	None	Hypnotic

- Compounds lacking Phase I metabolism with short elimination half-lives are preferred as hypnotics (but note nitrazepam, historically used as a hypnotic, has a very long half-life).

Clinical effects of Benzodiazepines

BDZs have anxiolytic, hypnotic, myorelaxant, anticonvulsant and anamnestic effects and impair psychomotor function

- Induction and maintenance of sleep
  - Shorter elimination half-life compounds are preferable.
  - Newer compounds (zolpidem, zopiclone and zaleplon) may have lower risks of dependence and withdrawal.
  - Very short half-life compounds (zaleplon) are only useful for sleep induction and not sleep maintenance.
- Treatment in anxiety disorders
  - Longer half-life drugs are preferable.
  - BDZs are effective in 'core' anxiety disorders; efficacy seems to be maintained for most patients with GAD and panic disorder, although some patients develop tolerance.
  - Have an earlier onset of effect than SSRIs which may be useful whilst waiting for SSRIs to become effective.
- Alcohol withdrawal and epilepsy/seizure termination
  - Longer half-life drugs indicated
- Other clinical uses
  - Premedication before anaesthesia and minor surgical procedures (sedation, anamnestic effect – short-to-intermediate half-life drugs indicated).
  - Muscle spasticity (longer half-life drugs indicated).

Adverse effects and safety of Benzodiazepines (Table 6.4)

The context of use determines whether some side effects (e.g. sedation and amnesia) are wanted or unwanted (see clinical effects)

- Reports of cleft lip and cleft palate after use in pregnancy in uncontrolled studies.
- Respiratory depression may occur in the newborn of mothers on BDZs. Developmental dysmorphism (as with foetal alcohol syndrome) has been reported, but maternal alcohol use a potential confounding factor.
- Epidemiological studies have suggested that BDZ may be a risk factor for subsequent development of cognitive impairment.

Table 6.4 Main adverse effects of benzodiazepines	
Frequency	Adverse effect
Common	Drowsiness, dizziness and psychomotor impairment
Occasional	Dry mouth, blurred vision, gastrointestinal upset, headache and increased risk of falls in the elderly
Rare	Amnesia, restlessness, disinhibition, skin rash, eosinophilia, respiratory arrest (parenteral administration), possible foetal developmental abnormalities and possible risk factor for cognitive impairment

- BDZs are relatively safe in overdose: Patients have survived taking more than 2 g of diazepam. Cognitive and psychomotor impairment can be detected for some weeks afterwards. Treatment of overdose involves the following:
  - Supportive therapy and gastric lavage if appropriate.
  - Dialysis is probably of limited value given the large volume of distribution of these drugs.
  - Flumazenil will counteract sedation but beware of its short half-life.

Tolerance to Benzodiazepines

- Increased rapid eye movement (REM) sleep amount and intensity (REM rebound) is one example of the development of tolerance to the effects of BDZ when used as a hypnotic:
  - BDZs reduce REM sleep from 25% to 10%–15% of total sleep time at night with tolerance occurring within about 2 weeks (REM% returns to normal).
  - Sudden discontinuation of BDZ leads to a rebound increase in REM sleep resulting in periods of waking through the night (can take up to 6 weeks to return to normal).
- Tolerance to different effects of BDZs not entirely clear – evidence suggests the following:
  - *Animals*: Tolerance occurs to sedation, ataxia, muscle relaxation and anticonvulsant effects but less clear for 'anxiolytic' effects.
  - *Humans*: Tolerance to sedation, anticonvulsant and EEG effects but less clear for psychomotor, anxiolytic and hypnotic effects.
- Cross-tolerance may occur to other BDZs and alcohol.
- The causes of tolerance with BDZs are not entirely clear but probably involve pharmacodynamic and cognitive/behavioural factors (see also Chapter 2).

Benzodiazepine withdrawal symptoms

- First fully described by Petursson and Lader in early 1980s: Had previously been recognised following prolonged, high-dose treatment, but they described it following shorter periods of standard doses
  - Probably affects 45% on cessation or dose reduction.
  - Personality variables have some predictive value: More common in a dependent personality.
- *Symptoms include*
  - Anxiety and anxiety-related (including mood and sleep disturbance, tremor, sweating, GI symptoms, muscle pains and fatigue)
  - Perceptual disturbance (including sensory hypersensitivity, sense of body sway or abnormal body sensations, depersonalisation and visual disturbance)
  - Rarely severe symptoms (major depression, psychosis and seizures)
- *Management of BDZ withdrawal*
  - Gradually decrease BDZ dose over 4–16 weeks.
  - Transfer to longer half-life drug, for example diazepam.
  - β-Blockers can reduce severity of symptoms but do not appear to improve outcome.
  - Monitor for increased alcohol consumption.
- Gradual dose reduction, brief psychological interventions and withdrawal with prescribing interventions can be effective in facilitating discontinuation of BDZs.

Benzodiazepines in clinical practice

- Reserve BDZs for patients with chronic, severe, distressing and disabling symptoms which have not responded to psychosocial management or to other psychological or pharmacological treatments.
- Use the lowest effective dose.
- Prescribe for brief periods in the generality of patients (although there is a role for longer-term treatment in a small minority of patients).
- Avoid 'repeat' prescriptions as far as possible.
- Warn patients about the possibility of tolerance, dependence and withdrawal symptoms.

Pregabalin

This is licensed for GAD in the European Union/United Kingdom but not in the United States.

Pharmacology of pregabalin

- A branched chain amino acid similar in structure to leucine and GABA.
- High affinity for $\alpha2\delta$ subunit of voltage-gated Ca^{2+} channels and believed to reduce the availability and effects of excitatory neurotransmitters, including glutamate.
- In spite of its name, it does not interact directly with GABA pathways.
- Absorbed rapidly after oral administration, requiring active transport with the L-type amino acid transporter 1 (LAT1), and achieves maximum plasma concentration within 1 h with a short half-life of about 6 h.
- Negligible hepatic metabolism and primarily eliminated unchanged by renal excretion.

Clinical efficacy of pregabalin

- Pregabalin has been shown to attenuate the activation of the left anterior insula and left amygdala in response to emotionally charged visual stimuli in healthy volunteers.
- Evidence in treating anxiety disorders is mainly in GAD and social phobia with efficacy demonstrated in
  - Acute treatment and relapse prevention
  - Augmentation after non-response to antidepressants in GAD
  - Symptomatic improvement in sleep, physical symptoms of anxiety and depressed mood
- Also licensed for the treatment of epilepsy, neuropathic pain and fibromyalgia.
- There is some evidence that it facilitates withdrawal from BDZ and related compounds.

Adverse effects of pregabalin

- Generally well tolerated
- Side effects include
  - Dizziness, vertigo and weight gain (significant in around 4% of patients)
  - Uncommonly peripheral oedema, worsened hepatic function and pleural effusion
- Serious complications with overdose are unusual but on case report of complete but transient atrioventricular block
- Dependence and abuse potential
  - Euphoria found in 1%–10% of patients in clinical trials
  - Reports of pregabalin abuse (often in those with a history of abuse of other medications)
- Discontinuation symptoms after abrupt withdrawal; more prominent with higher doses but less prominent than with BDZs.

5-HT$_{1A}$ receptor agonists (azapirones)

- Buspirone (5-HT$_{1A}$ receptor partial agonist) became available in mid-1980s: Tandospirone is available in some Asian countries. Others have been developed (ipsapirone and gepirone) but are not available for clinical use.

Pharmacology of buspirone

- Buspirone initially stimulates somatodendritic 5-HT$_{1A}$ autoreceptors, causing decreased 5-HT neuronal firing and terminal release. Repeated treatment desensitises the autoreceptor and reinstates normal of 5-HT neuronal firing and release. This, together with direct postsynaptic 5-HT$_{1A}$ receptor stimulation, may lead to overall increase in 5-HT$_{1A}$ function. This is a similar mechanism to that seen with SSRIs (see Chapter 4, Figure 4.1).
- Short elimination half-life (3 h) means multiple daily dosing is required.
- The active metabolite 1-(2-pyrimidinyl)piperazine (1-PP, an α_2 antagonist) may contribute to efficacy.

Clinical effiacy of buspirone

- Effective in GAD, but not in panic disorder or social phobia. No consistent evidence in treatment of other anxiety disorders
- Some evidence for greater efficacy if patients without previous exposure to BDZs
- May reduce depressive symptoms (also evidence for modest efficacy in treating major depression)
- Ineffective as augmenting agent for SSRIs in depressive and anxiety disorders
- Appear less effective than BDZs and takes longer to act so of little use in treating acute anxiety

Adverse effects of buspirone

- Include nausea, dizziness and headache; akathisia can rarely occur with higher doses
- No evidence of a withdrawal syndrome, and no interaction with alcohol

Antidepressants (see also Chapter 4)

- SSRIs are now widely viewed as first line for the pharmacological treatment of anxiety disorders and have the most extensive evidence base (Table 6.5).

Table 6.5 Summary of treatments with placebo-controlled randomised controlled trial evidence for efficacy in the pharmacological treatment of anxiety-related disorders

	GAD	Panic disorder	Social phobia	PTSD	OCD
Acute treatment	SSRIs[a] SNRIs[a] Imipramine Trazodone Vortioxetine Agomelatine BDZs[a] Pregabalin Buspirone Trifluoperazine Quetiapine Hydroxyzine	SSRIs[a] Venlafaxine Reboxetine TCAs[a] Phenelzine BDZs[a] Gabapentin Valproate	SSRIs[a] Venlafaxine MAOI[a] (Mirtazapine) BDZs[a] Gabapentin Pregabalin Olanzapine	SSRIs[a] Venlafaxine (TCAs[a]) (Mirtazapine) (Nefazodone) (Phenelzine) (Atypical antipsy- chotics) (Topiramate)	SSRIs[a] Clomip- ramine
Relapse pre-vention	SSRIs[a] TCAs[a] Vortioxetine Agomelatine Pregabalin Quetiapine	SSRIs[a] Venlafaxine Imipramine	SSRIs[a] Clonazepam Pregabalin	SSRIs[a]	SSRIs[a]
Augmen-tation after non-response	Pregabalin Atypical antipsy- chotics[a]	Pindolol	—	Prazosin Olanzapine (Risperidone)	Haloperidol Atypical antipsy- chotics[a] $5\text{-}HT_3$ antagonists[a] Topiramate Lamotrigine

Source: Adapted from Baldwin B et al., *J Psychopharmacol* 2014; 28: 403. BAP guidelines.

[a] More than one drug within class but specific drugs vary between disorders; () inconsistent or equivocal efficacy: see Baldwin et al. (2014) BAP guidelines for details.

- Historical background
  - TCAs, although used for many years to treat anxiety disorders, were not tested in large randomised controlled trials (RCTs) until the 1970s.
  - The efficacy of imipramine against panic attacks was used to support arguments for the panic disorder being a distinct condition (in the erroneous belief that panic disorder did not respond to BDZ).
  - Clomipramine was the first drug treatment demonstrated to be of benefit for OCD.
  - MAOIs have traditionally been used in 'atypical depression', which historically includes mild/moderate depressive states with a large anxiety component. They have possible greater efficacy than imipramine, but have not been compared with SSRIs for this indication.
  - More recently, extensive RCTs with SSRIs and SNRIs have been carried out.
- Efficacy in anxiety disorders is probably related to their effects on 5-HT neurotransmission (effects on NA function may also contribute).
- See Chapter 4 for details of antidepressants and their adverse effects.

Efficacy of antidepressants (Table 6.5)

- As a class, SSRIs have proven efficacy across the range of anxiety disorders, although not all SSRIs have published evidence in all disorders.
- SNRIs and TCAs also appear to have a broad efficacy across disorders, but the evidence base is less complete than for SSRIs.
- Only antidepressants inhibiting 5-HT reuptake (SSRIs and clomipramine) have been shown to be effective in OCD, but evidence is lacking for many serotonergic drugs with the same (e.g. SNRIs) or different (e.g. mirtazapine) mechanism of action.
- Other antidepressants such as MAOIs, mirtazapine, reboxetine, agomelatine and vortioxetine have shown efficacy in some anxiety disorders (Table 6.5).

Antidepressants in clinical practice

- SSRIs are recommended first-line pharmacological treatment for anxiety disorders.
- Serotonergic TCAs are recommended second-line treatments in panic disorder (clomipramine and imipramine) and OCD (clomipramine).
- In the first 2 weeks of treatment with an SSRI, anxiety symptoms may worsen, but the incidence, clinical features, aetiology and optimal management of this 'activation syndrome' are all poorly characterised.
- A response to acute treatment should be followed by longer-term treatment: The optimal duration of continuation treatment is uncertain.

- Once continuation treatment is complete, it may be reasonable to steadily reduce dosage but the optimal duration of this tapering period is uncertain.

Antipsychotic drugs (see Chapter 3)

- Antipsychotics, particularly lower potency sedative drugs, have traditionally been used clinically as adjunctive therapy for severe and treatment-resistant anxiety disorders.
- There have been relatively few clinical trials, most small and not placebo controlled.
- RCTs provide evidence of efficacy for (Table 6.5)
  - Second-generation (atypical) antipsychotic augmentation of SSRIs in PTSD
  - First- and second-generation antipsychotic augmentation of SSRIs in OCD
  - Quetiapine and trifluoperazine monotherapy in GAD
  - Olanzapine in social phobia
  - Olanzapine augmentation of fluoxetine in GAD
- May be useful for short-term use in reducing anxiety/agitation associated with severe depressive disorder in addition to their use as augmenting agents (see Chapter 4).
- Adverse effects potentially limit the usefulness of antipsychotics for anxiety disorders (EPSE and tardive dyskinesia from first-generation drugs, metabolic syndrome with second-generation drugs).
- Current role is in careful augmentation treatment trials in GAD, OCD and PTSD responding poorly to other treatments.

β-Adrenoceptor antagonists ('β-blockers')

- *Efficacy*
  - Early exploratory trials demonstrated a reduction in some physical anxiety symptoms due to peripheral blockade β-adrenoceptors.
  - Anxiety symptoms associated with thyrotoxicosis were shown to reduce with β-blocker treatment: It is unclear whether this is mainly through β_1- or β_2-adrenoceptors.
  - Numerous small studies, some placebo controlled, show benefit in situational/performance anxiety.
  - β-Blockers lack effect in ameliorating psychological symptoms in anxiety disorders.
  - They may attenuate the severity of BDZ withdrawal symptoms.
- *Adverse effects include*
  - Hypotension, bradycardia and excessive dreaming
  - Bronchospasm and cardiac failure in patients with asthma and cardiac disease
  - Possible depression of mood (inconsistent evidence)

- *Indications*
  - Anxiety symptoms in patients with situational/performance anxiety.
  - Some GAD/panic disorder patients with prominent physiological symptoms of anxiety.
  - Akathisia and lithium-induced fine tremor (not toxicity).

Other pharmacological treatments

- *Selective orexin (hypocretin) receptor antagonists* have potential efficacy in sleep disorders (suvorexant approved for treatment of insomnia by the USA FDA in 2014) and investigation as potential anxiolytics is warranted.
- *Hydroxyzine* (antihistamine) has been shown to have short-term efficacy in GAD.
- Some *anticonvulsants* have efficacy in some anxiety disorders (Table 6.5).
- *CCK antagonists* have not shown evidence for efficacy in clinical trials, probably related to poor CNS bioavailability.
- *Neurokinin (NK, substance P) receptor antagonists* have been investigated based on effects in laboratory animals, but evidence from clinical trials has been inconsistent and disappointing.
- Some *'complementary treatments'* may have beneficial effects in some patients with anxiety symptoms: The best evidence is for lavender oil preparations in patients with GAD.

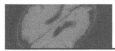

Principles of drug treatment of anxiety disorders

- Many authorities recommend psychological treatments initially for anxiety disorders. Most patients who meet full diagnostic criteria for an anxiety disorder derive benefit from psychological or pharmacological treatment.
- Accurate diagnosis of the type of anxiety disorder enables identification of the pharmacological treatments with the best evidence-base.
- SSRIs are general first-line treatment, but comorbidity, concomitant medication and treatment history influence treatment decisions; for example, antidepressants rather than BDZ or other anxiolytics are indicated for comorbid depressive symptoms of moderate or greater severity.
- For most disorders, treatment trials of up to 12 weeks are needed to assess benefit, this may be shorter for GAD.

- Treatment should be continued for at least 6 months after acute treatment, longer for GAD (18 months).
- Add psychological treatment (usually CBT) for insufficient response, or to reduce the risk of relapse.
- For insufficient response, after considering dose increase (especially panic disorder and OCD), options are to switch to an alternative effective treatment, or augment (especially OCD and PTSD) (Table 6.5).

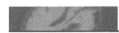

Acknowledgement

This is an update and revision of the third edition chapter by Stephen J Cooper.

Bibliography

Guidelines

Baldwin DS, Anderson IM, Nutt DJ et al. Evidence-based pharmacological treatment of anxiety disorders, post-traumatic stress disorder and obsessive-compulsive disorder: A revision of the 2005 guidelines from the British Association for Psychopharmacology. *J Psychopharmacol.* 2014; 28: 403–439. http://www.bap.org.uk/pdfs/AnxietyGuidelines2014.pdf.

Bandelow B, Zohar J, Hollander E et al. World Federation of Societies of Biological Psychiatry (WFSBP) guidelines for the pharmacological treatment of anxiety, obsessive-compulsive and post-traumatic stress disorders – First revision. *World J Biol Psychiatry.* 2008; 9: 248–312.

National Institute for Health and Care Excellence. Guidance on the use of zaleplon, zolpidem and zopiclone for the short-term management of insomnia. *NICE Technology Appraisal Guidance 77.* 2004; http://www.nice.org.uk/guidance/ta77.

National Institute for Health and Care Excellence. Obsessive-compulsive disorder: Core interventions in the treatment of obsessive compulsive disorder and body dysmorphic disorder. *NICE Clinical Guideline 31.* 2005; http://www.nice.org.uk/guidance/cg31.

National Institute for Health and Care Excellence. Post-traumatic stress disorder (PTSD): The management of PTSD in adults and children in primary and secondary care. *NICE Clinical Guideline 26.* 2005; http://www.nice.org.uk/guidance/cg26.

National Institute for Health and Care Excellence. Generalised anxiety disorder and panic disorder (with or without agoraphobia) in adults: Management in primary, secondary and community care. *NICE Clinical Guideline 113.* 2011; http://www.nice.org.uk/guidance/cg113.

National Institute for Health and Care Excellence. Social anxiety disorder: Recognition, assessment and treatment. *NICE Clinical Guideline 159.* 2013; http://www.nice.org.uk/guidance/cg159.

Wilson SJ, Nutt DJ, Alford C et al. British Association for Psychopharmacology consensus statement on evidence-based treatment of insomnia, parasomnias and circadian rhythm disorders. *J Psychopharmacol.* 2010; 24: 1577–1601. http://www.bap.org.uk/pdfs/BAP_Sleep_Guidelines.pdf.

Key references

Baldwin DS, Aitchison K, Bateson A et al. Benzodiazepines: Risks and benefits. A reconsideration. *J Psychopharmacol.* 2013; 27: 967–971. http://www.bap.org.uk/pdfs/Benzodiazepines_Guidelines_2013.pdf.

Baldwin DS, Ajel K, Masdrakis VG et al. Pregabalin for the treatment of generalized anxiety disorder: An update. *Neuropsychiatr Dis Treat.* 2013b; 9: 883–892.

Baldwin DS, Kosky N. Off-label prescribing in psychiatric practice. *Adv Psychiat Treat.* 2007; 13: 414–422.

Billioti de Gage S, Moride Y, Ducruet T et al. Benzodiazepine use and risk of Alzheimer's disease: Case control study. *BMJ.* 2014; 349: g5205.

Gould RL, Coulson MC, Patel N et al. Interventions for reducing benzodiazepine use in older people: Meta-analysis of randomised controlled trials. *Br J Psychiatry.* 2014; 204: 98–107.

Hou R, Baldwin DS. A neuroimmunological perspective on anxiety disorders. *Hum Psychopharmacol.* 2012; 27: 6–14.

Parr JM, Kavanagh DJ, Cahill L et al. Effectiveness of current treatment approaches for benzodiazepine discontinuation: A meta-analysis. *Addiction.* 2009; 104: 13–24.

Further reading

Allgulander C. History and current status of sedative-hypnotic drug use and abuse (review article). *Acta Psych. Scand.* 1986; 73: 465–478.

Baldwin D, Leonard B. *Anxiety Disorders.* Basel, Switzerland: Karger, 2013.

Bandelow B, Domschke K, Baldwin D. *Panic Disorder and Agoraphobia.* Oxford, UK: Oxford University Press, 2014.

Gould RL, Coulson MC, Patel N et al. Interventions for reducing benzodiazepine use in older people: Meta-analysis of randomised controlled trials. *Br J Psychiatry.* 2014; 204: 98–107.

Jacobson LH, Callander GE, Hoyer D. Suvorexant for the treatment of insomnia. *Exp Rev Clin Pharmacol.* 2014; 7: 711–730.

Miller R. *Drugged, The Science and Culture Behind Psychotropic Drugs.* Oxford, UK: Oxford University Press, 2014.

Montgomery S, Baldwin D. *Clinicians Manual on Generalized Anxiety Disorder.* London, UK: Current Medicine Group, 2006.

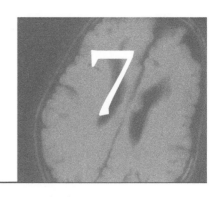

Drugs of abuse

Anne Lingford-Hughes and Mark Daglish

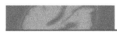 ## Why take drugs?

- For pleasure, to get a 'rush', euphoria, i.e., for positive reinforcement or reward
- Anxiolytic or to overcome withdrawal, that is, negative reinforcement
- Because their use cannot be controlled, overwhelming urge, compulsion

The faster the onset of the drug effects, the better the 'rush':

Slow					Fast
Chewing tobacco	→		Snuff	→	Cigarettes
Coca leaves	→	Coca paste	→ Cocaine	→	Crack cocaine
Methadone	→	Morphine	→ Snorted heroin	→	Intravenous heroin

 ## History

- The pattern of drug use changes with time depending on what is available, the social context and how much it costs.
- Many drugs, which are now considered 'addictive', were often introduced for medical purposes.
- *Alcohol*
  - Evidence of fermentation processes occurring approximately 7000 years ago.
  - Currently is the mostly widely used legal drug and relative cost is decreasing.

- *Opioids*
  - Opium has been used medically since ancient times.
  - Morphine was isolated in 1805.
  - Methadone was first synthesised in Germany during World War II.
- *Stimulants*
  - *Amfetamine (amphetamine)* was synthesised in the late 1880s for therapeutic purposes.
  - Cocaine alkaloid was first isolated in 1860 and used as a local anaesthetic.
  - Methamphetamine (derivative of amphetamine) is increasingly used in the United States, United Kingdom and other countries.
- *Cannabis*
  - Its effects have been documented for many centuries.
  - Its non-medical use, for its hedonic properties, began in the early nineteenth century in Europe.
- *Hallucinogens*, include both natural (psilocybin) and synthetic (lysergic acid diethylamide [LSD]) compounds
  - Hallucinogenic powers of LSD were discovered when it was accidentally absorbed in 1943. In the 1950s, the term 'psychedelic' was coined.
  - Use of psychedelic drugs predominated in the 1960s.
- *Tobacco*, a native plant of the American continent
  - Believed to have been first used in the first century.
  - Smoked in Europe from around the end of the fifteenth century.
- 'Novel psychoactive substances', multiple series of compounds (including so-called legal highs) designed and synthesised to mimic other drugs of abuse
  - Large increase in number of different substances available on the Internet (in Europe, ~40 new compounds/year)
  - Many have unknown constituents with unknown pharmacological properties

In conceptualising the recreational use/misuse of drugs, different models have been applied:

- Medical (disease model)
- Psychological (learning theory)
- Philosophical/moral

Legal issues (United Kingdom)

- The Misuse of Drugs Act 1971 relates to the manufacture, supply and possession of 'controlled drugs'. Drugs are ascribed to one of three classes based on the perceived harmfulness when they are misused;

the penalties are set accordingly (see the British National Formulary [BNF] for the complete listing, and check for updates):

- *Class A* includes cannabinol (except where contained in cannabis or cannabis resin), cocaine, diamorphine (heroin), dipipanone, lysergide (LSD), methadone, methylenedioxymethamphetamine (MDMA or Ecstasy), morphine, opium, oxycodone, pethidine, phencyclidine, psilocin and class B substances when prepared for injection.
- *Class B* includes oral amphetamines, barbiturates, cannabis and cannabis resin, codeine, methamphetamine and pentazocine.
- *Class C* includes buprenorphine (Bup), diethylpropion, khat (from July 2013), mazindol, meprobamate, pemoline, pipradrol, most benzodiazepines (BDZs), androgenic and anabolic steroids, clenbuterol and certain drugs related to the amphetamines such as benzphetamine and chlorphentermine.
- *Temporary class drug order (2011)* set up for any new psychoactive substance that is raising sufficient concern for government to act quickly to protect the public, for example benzofuran, 25I-NBOMe (also called Cimbi-5, 25I, a substituted phenylethylamine psychedelic).

- At the time of publication the UK government is proposing blanket legislation to ban novel psychoactive substances (so called 'legal highs').
- Prescribing issues – see the British National Formulary:
  - For regulations related to prescribing of controlled drugs
  - For appropriate guidelines (see also BAP and NICE) regarding information about prescribing, current indications, side effects, cautions and contraindications

Scientific background

- Drugs of abuse increase DA concentration in the nucleus accumbens (NAcc) of the mesolimbic system, but to varying magnitude, for example small with opioids (Figure 7.1).
- Increase in DA function is key in mediating positive reinforcement:
  - DA increased by cocaine, amphetamine, alcohol, opiates, nicotine and cannabinoids (Figure 7.1).
  - BDZs are the only drugs of abuse not shown to significantly increase DA.
- NAcc
  - Has high levels of D_3 receptors.
  - DA is released here and, in the amygdala, is also involved in learning associations, that is, draws attention to certain significant events.
- Reduced DA concentrations are seen in withdrawal states and are likely to be associated with depression, irritability and dysphoria.

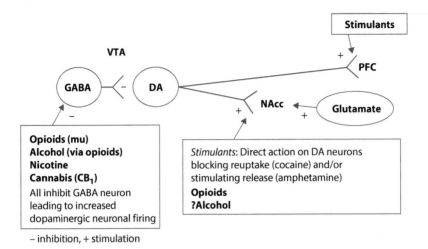

Figure 7.1 The DA reinforcement pathway. DA neurons in the VTA project to mesolimbic areas (including NAcc) and prefrontal cortex (PFC). GABA neurons in the VTA inhibit DA neuronal firing and can be inhibited by drugs such as opioids through μ-receptors and cannabinoids through CB₁ receptors. This results in disinhibition (activation) of the DA neurons and increased release of DA in NAcc (and PFC). Stimulant drugs act directly on DA neurons in the NAcc and PFC.

- Sensitisation (a progressive increase in an effect of a drug with repeated administration; see Chapter 2) is associated with stimulant abuse.
- DA is indirectly modulated by
  - Opioid and GABA neurons (Figure 7.1).
  - These connections underpin the pharmacological basis for GABA_B agonists', and opioid antagonists', efficacy in the treatment of alcohol dependence.

Alcohol

Neuropharmacology

There is no 'alcohol receptor' as such. Alcohol primarily modulates ion channel function (GABA–BDZ, N-methyl-D-aspartate [NMDA], 5-HT$_3$ receptors). The effect on different neurotransmitter systems is described in the following sections.

Alcohol and GABA function

- Alcohol mediates many of its actions through modulating GABA function; it is an agonist at GABA–BDZ receptors (see Chapter 1 for details of GABA receptors).
- Different subunits of the receptor confer different alcohol sensitivities:
  - Recently α_5-containing receptors have been shown to be involved with alcohol reinforcement.
  - Varied individual sensitivity is a possible mechanism of vulnerability to alcoholism.
- Chronic ethanol exposure is associated with
  - Reduced GABA–BDZ receptor function and reduced levels of specific receptor subunits leading to tolerance.
  - This interaction underlies the cross-tolerance between alcohol and BDZ.
- In alcohol dependence, stimulation of $GABA_B$ receptors with agonists (e.g. baclofen; see Treatment of alcohol dependence section) reduces the risk of relapse.

Alcohol and glutamate function

- Alcohol is an NMDA antagonist causing decreased Ca^{2+} influx into neurons and decreased excitability (see Chapter 1). This may account for effects on memory, for example amnesia (blackouts).
- Chronic ethanol exposure increases NMDA receptor function which leads in withdrawal to a hyperexcitable state. This is probably the mechanism underlying seizures and brain damage through excitatory neurotoxicity.

Alcohol and monoamine function

Dopamine:

- Reduced DA responses are seen in patients with alcoholism.
- These reduced responses may predict relapse and be associated with depressive symptomatology – dysphoria, irritability and restlessness.
- Association reported in some groups of alcoholism with a D_2 receptor polymorphism.
- D_2 receptor-deficient mice show marked aversion to alcohol.
- PET studies show reduced levels of $D_{2/3}$ receptors in abstinent alcoholism; however, recent study showed no change in D_3 receptors in the brain except for increased levels in the hypothalamus.

Noradrenaline:

▪ Increased activity may occur in alcohol withdrawal; however, lofexidine (α_2-adrenoceptor agonist) does not symptomatically improve alcohol withdrawal.

Serotonin:

▪ Low levels of 5-HT particularly associated with *type II alcoholism* (early onset, high impulsivity, positive family history of alcoholism, male predominance).
▪ Increased 5-HT function may
   – Be associated with *type I alcoholism* (later onset, mixed gender, anxious)
   – Lead to craving
   – Increase anxiety
▪ 5-HT is implicated in many disorders which coexist with alcoholism: Depression/suicide, anxiety disorders and bulimia nervosa.

Alcohol and other receptors

▪ Opioids: See the section on 'Scientific background' section.
▪ Peptides such as neuropeptide Y, NK1 and gut hormones such as ghrelin are currently being studied.

Neurochemistry of alcohol withdrawal

Alcohol withdrawal is associated with:

▪ *Increased activity in*:
   – NDMA receptors
   – L-Subtype of Ca^{2+} channels

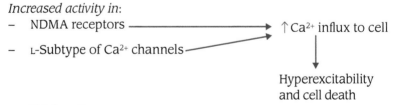

$\uparrow Ca^{2+}$ influx to cell

Hyperexcitability and cell death

   – NA function
▪ *Decreases in*:
   – GABA function.
   – Mg^{2+} inhibition of the NMDA receptor (thereby increasing NMDA function).
   – DA function.

Treatment of alcohol withdrawal

- BDZs to increase GABA function.
- Vitamins (thiamine [B_1], B complex) as dependent drinkers are likely to be vitamin (especially thiamine) deficient due to poor diet and poor absorption. Parenteral thiamine must be given if patient is at risk of Wernicke's encephalopathy as poorly absorbed orally (caution as anaphylaxis is a rare but recognised risk). If the oral preparation is appropriate, give doses more frequently to maximise absorption.
- Carbamazepine has shown efficacy and may be an alternative if BDZs contraindicated or ineffective.

Neurochemistry related to drugs used for alcohol dependence

See Table 7.1.

Treatment of alcohol dependence

- A variety of drugs have been used in the treatment of alcohol dependence with varying success.
- Comorbid psychiatric disorders may require treatment, but ideally patients should not be started on psychotropic drugs until it is clear which symptoms are alcohol related, for example wait 2–3 weeks following abstinence from alcohol before using antidepressants to treat depression, as symptoms may subside spontaneously.

Table 7.1 Neurochemistry related to medications that have been used in the treatment of alcoholism

Neurochemistry	Pharmacology
Dopamine	Agonist (bromocriptine)
	Antagonist (D_1, D_2)
Serotonin	Reuptake inhibitors (SSRIs)
	Antagonist: 5-HT_3 (ondansetron)
	Partial agonist: 5-HT_{1A} (buspirone)
Opioid	Antagonist (naltrexone, nalmefene)
GABA	Topiramate, baclofen
Glutamate (NMDA)	Acamprosate

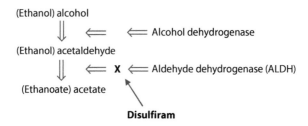

Figure 7.2   Disulfiram inhibits the metabolism of acetaldehyde to acetate.

Disulfiram

- Disulfiram inhibits aldehyde dehydrogenase (Figure 7.2).
- This leads to a build-up of acetaldehyde (ethanol) if alcohol is consumed causing adverse effects:
  - Nausea and vomiting
  - Flushing
  - Palpitations
  - Headache
  - Hypotension
- Disulfiram also inhibits dopamine-β-hydroxylase leading to an increase in DA and reduction in NA in the brain; however, it is unclear if this is related to its efficacy.
- Contraindications are psychosis, severe liver or cardiac disease and epilepsy.
- Supervision or witnessed consumption is associated with improved outcome.

Acamprosate

- A taurine derivative.
- Its exact pharmacology is still not clear, but it is a functional antagonist (see Chapter 2) of glutamate NMDA receptor function, possibly through effect on AMPA receptors.
- Approximately doubles abstinence rates to about 20%–40% and also increases 'time to first drink'.
- May reduce likelihood of an episode of drinking becoming a relapse.
- Adverse effects generally mild: GI disturbance.
- Described as 'anti-craving' (contentious).
- Contraindicated if severe liver damage.
- There are no clear predictors of efficacy.

Opioid antagonists

- Naltrexone (non-selective μ, κ and δ antagonist): In alcohol dependence it
  - Reduces craving
  - Reduces lapse/relapse rate
  - Is contraindicated in acute hepatitis or severe liver failure
- Nalmefene (μ antagonist and partial κ agonist): Currently licensed for those who are dependent, engaged with psychosocial treatment, need to reduce consumption but unable to do so and do not need detoxification (i.e. start when drinking and can take 'as needed').

Topiramate (see also Chapter 5)

- Anticonvulsant drug recently reported to improve drinking behaviour (reduced drinking days, greater abstinence rates) in alcohol-dependent subjects
- Given when still actively drinking but in an abstinence-focused treatment plan

Baclofen

- $GABA_B$ agonist reported to increase abstinence rates in alcohol-dependent patients who want abstinence.
- May be particularly effective in those with significant anxiety.
- Generally well tolerated, sedation most common and particularly with alcohol.
- Current trials are examining optimal dose.

Treatment of comorbidity

Address alcohol consumption, including consideration of medication described earlier.

Depression

- Depressive symptoms and disorder are common and as likely to precede alcohol abuse as to be a consequence of it.
- Persistent depressive symptoms following withdrawal from alcohol should be treated (see Chapter 4).
- Trials of antidepressants in alcohol disorder and depression (TCAs and SSRIs) do not consistently show efficacy:
  - Meta-analyses suggest that antidepressants (TCA, SSRI) alone have limited efficacy in improving mood or drinking behaviour.

- Use of SSRIs in non-depressed type II alcohol dependence (mostly men, onset <25 years, more severely dependent, stronger genetic basis, associated with impulsive and aggressive traits) either results in no improvement or may worsen outcome.
- Limited evidence is available for newer antidepressants.

Anxiety

- As with depression, anxiety may be a cause, and a consequence, of alcohol abuse.
- Panic attacks and generalised anxiety disorder (GAD) can emerge from alcohol dependence.
- Treatment of comorbid anxiety disorders has not been studied to the same extent as for depression.
- BDZs should rarely be used due to their addictive potential.
- Buspirone (5-HT$_{1A}$ partial agonist) has been shown to reduce anxiety and drinking behaviour.
- Antidepressants have been shown to have some benefit in reducing panic attacks in alcoholic subjects.

Schizophrenia

- Fourfold increase of alcoholism in schizophrenia; more common than drug misuse (excluding nicotine dependence).
- Evidence that substance misuse increases risk of psychotic relapse even with good antipsychotic adherence.
- Recent studies do not show clear benefit of atypical over typical antipsychotics, except possibly for clozapine, which has been reported to be associated with less substance misuse (although there are no prospective trials).
- High serum prolactin, secondary to DA blockade by antipsychotics, is associated with higher alcohol consumption in people with schizophrenia.

Bipolar disorder

- Twelvefold increase risk of mania in males with alcoholism.
- Challenging to manage and with limited evidence for optimal pharmacotherapy; valproate may improve outcome.
- There is evidence showing efficacy of naltrexone.

Opiates/opioids

The term 'opiates' refers to natural substances derived from the opium poppy (e.g. morphine, codeine) and 'opioids' to all, including semisynthetic (e.g. heroin [diamorphine] and dihydrocodeine) and synthetic (e.g. methadone) compounds.

- Opioids act as agonists at
  - μ (mu) receptors – Analgesia, euphoria, positive reinforcement, respiratory depression. High affinity binding for enkephalins and β-endorphin; morphine, codeine, and methadone bind to the μ-receptor.
  - κ (kappa) receptors – Dysphoria, sedation, analgesia. Dynorphins are the endogenous ligands.
  - δ (delta) receptors – Analgesia and possibly seizures. Enkephalins are the endogenous ligands.
  - NB σ (sigma) receptors were originally thought to be opioid receptors but are now classified separately.
- *Acute effects*: Miosis, euphoria, tranquillity, drowsiness, itching, nausea, respiratory depression.
- *Chronic effects*: Anhedonia, depression, insomnia, hyperprolactinaemia, constipation, dependence.
- Mechanism of tolerance to opioids is not well understood with variability depending on effect (e.g. tolerance to euphoria, but not to their impact on pupillary muscles). No clear changes in opioid receptor numbers reported, suggesting intracellular changes or alterations in other systems.

Opioid withdrawal

- *Symptoms*
  - Mydriasis, diarrhoea, dysphoria, insomnia, restlessness, 'craving'.
  - Associated with increased NA function: Tachycardia, sweating, piloerection, rhinorrhoea, shivering
- Opioid withdrawal is associated with increased NA function due to opioid effects in the locus coeruleus:
  - Acute effects of opioids are to inhibit cAMP and reduce NA neuronal firing.
  - With chronic exposure, compensatory upregulation of cAMP occurs, with an increase in NA neuronal 'tone' which is revealed on withdrawal of opioids.
- *Treatment*
  - Opioid substitute therapy
  - Symptomatic treatment for gastrointestinal disturbance, insomnia, muscle aches
  - Lofexidine, an α_2 agonist, to reduce NA-related symptoms (side effects: Sedation, hypotension)
- *Relapse prevention*: Following successful withdrawal from opioids, loss of tolerance leads to a high risk of fatal respiratory overdose with resumed use. Therefore, a detailed relapse plan with appropriate after care is prior to withdrawal.

Substitute therapies in opioid addiction

Principle: Use drugs with a longer half-life than 'street' opioids (Figure 7.3).

Methadone

- Full μ opioid agonist
- $t_{1/2}$ = approx. 36 h with single dose but reduces to approx. 24 h with regular use due to induction of CYP3A4
- Widely used in maintenance and slow outpatient withdrawal
- Risk of prolonged QTc at higher doses

Buprenorphine

- Partial agonist at μ opioid receptor; it has a reduced risk of fatal respiratory depression.
- Antagonist at κ opioid receptor, which may be why buprenorphine is less likely to cause dysphoria.
- $t_{1/2}$ > 24 h.

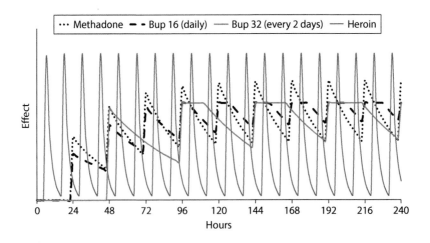

Figure 7.3 Pharmacology of opioid substitute therapy. Methadone is a relatively long-acting full agonist and Bup, a long-acting partial agonist that can be given daily or every other day (every 2 days). Their use avoids the 'highs' alternating with 'lows' associated with heroin (diamorphine).

- Longer $t_{1/2}$ and partial agonists make the withdrawal syndrome less severe.
- Safer than full agonists and reduces the effect of additional full (e.g. 'street') opioid agonists by blocking their effects (see Chapter 2 for discussion about partial agonists).
- Due to lower maximal effect, it can be given in larger doses, less frequently.
- Combined preparation with naloxone (non-orally absorbed opioid antagonist) used to reduce incidence of recreational iv use.

Naltrexone

- Oral non-selective opioid antagonist which blocks acute opioid effects.
- Long-acting (active metabolite gives effective $t_{1/2}$ of 96 h).
- Used to prevent relapse in drug-free subjects.
- Good compliance and monitoring are associated with better outcome.
- Most common side effects are gastrointestinal.

 **Stimulants**

Cocaine

- 'Crack' is the free base of cocaine and can be smoked, inhaled or injected giving a faster rate of onset than cocaine (snorted).
- Cocaine inhibits reuptake of DA (most important), 5-HT and NA, and is a Na^+ channel blocker (local anaesthetic, cardiac arrhythmias).
- *Pharmacokinetics of delivery important*: Cocaine 'rush' intensity due to fast uptake.
- *Acute effects*: Euphoria (related to DA transporter blockade), confusion, psychosis, increased blood pressure/pulse (can result in stroke, seizure), formication and then a 'crash' (see the following text).
- *Chronic effects*: Paranoia, psychosis, anorexia, depression.
- *Complex adaptation to chronic use*: Reduced dopaminergic function which may be partially reversible with abstinence, variable effect on D_1, D_2 receptor numbers/function.
- Withdrawal 'crash'
  - Depression, anxiety, hypersomnia, anergia.
  - Treatment with antidepressants (desipramine) is not thought to be effective in preventing this acute 'crash'.

Pharmacotherapy for cocaine addiction in development

- Vaccines
- Drugs such as disulfiram, baclofen and modafinil are under investigation

Amfetamine (amphetamine)

- Inhibits DA reuptake and also stimulates DA release
- Similar effects to cocaine
- Generally taken in pill form, can be injected

Methamfetamine (methamphetamine)

- Similar action to amphetamine in increasing DA through stimulating release and blocking reuptake.
- 'High' lasts much longer, 6–8 h compared with the brief high from cocaine.
- Can be taken orally, snorted, smoked and injected.
- Growing concerns about its neurotoxicity, which is likely to involve oxidative stress.

Khat (*Catha edulis*)

- Active ingredient is cathinone, with similar effects to amphetamine but much less strong.
- The fresh leaves of the khat plant are chewed.
- Currently used primarily by people from Horn of Africa and Yemen.

Synthetic cathinones

- Amphetamine-like synthetic compounds related to cathinone (see Khat).
- Multiple and changing variants sold under changing brand names (e.g. 3,4-methylenedioxypyrovalerone [MDPV], mephedrone).
- Pharmacology unclear but effects suggest DA and 5-HT reuptake inhibition.
- Have been associated with 'excited delirium' toxic states acutely.
- Consult European Monitoring Centre for Drugs and Drug Addiction website for up-to-date information on this rapidly changing scene (see Further reading).

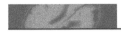 **Hallucinogens**

Glutamate (NMDA) receptor antagonists

Phencyclidine (PCP)

- *Acute effects*
  - Delusions, paranoia, disordered thinking (schizophrenic-like), illusions/hallucinations
  - Increased blood pressure/pulse
- *Chronic effects*
  - Cognitive impairment, depression
  - Weight loss

Ketamine

- Used as an anaesthetic agent and analgesic and there is current interest in its rapid antidepressant efficacy. It is abused as a 'club drug'.
- Can be injected or snorted.
- *Similar effects to PCP*: Prominent dissociative effects, dream-like states and hallucinations ('K-hole').
- Other effects include severe abdominal pain ('K-cramps') and in chronic use painful interstitial cystitis (which may require surgery), colitis and hepatitis.

Lysergic acid diethylamide

- Primary effect is via the serotonergic system (5-HT_{2A} agonist).
- *Acute effects* (*'trip'*): Mood swings, delusions, synaesthesia (e.g. hearing colours), panic, increased blood pressure/pulse.
- *Later effects*: 'Flashbacks', recurrence of unpleasant acute effects.

 **Enactogens**

- Produce experiences of emotional communion and relatedness, also known as empathogens
- *Prototype*: MDMA (Ecstasy)
- Stimulant/hallucinogenic depending on contents of the tablet
- *Derivatives*: Methylenedioxyamphetamine (MDA, Adam), methylenedioxyethylamphetamine (MDEA, Eve)
- 5-HT neurotoxin (at dorsal raphe nucleus) leading to
  - *In animal studies*: Loss of 5-HT neurons, 5-HT transporters, decreased 5-HIAA (5-HT metabolite) in CSF.
  - *Toxicity*: MDA > MDMA > MDEA.
  - Neurotoxicity of MDMA in humans is not clear.

- *Acute effects*: Empathy, increased blood pressure/pulse, dehydration, renal/heart failure, increased body temperature (greater with dancing), teeth clenching, reduced appetite
- *After-effects*: Midweek blues/depression, disordered sleep, presumed to be due to monoamine depletion
- *Chronic effects*: Memory impairment, depression
- Use associated with flashbacks, psychosis, depression, anxiety

 ## Nicotine

- Stimulant.
- Primary site of action is the nicotinic ACh receptor.
- Increases DA release in NAcc by increasing firing of ventral tegmental area (VTA) DA neurons.
- Tolerance is associated with receptor desensitisation and a compensatory upregulation of nicotinic receptors.
- Receptor desensitisation can lessen overnight and hence the first cigarette of the day has the greatest effect.
- Smoking associated with respiratory problems, many cancers and cardiovascular disease.
- While smoking is associated with depression and anxiety, nicotine appears to alleviate depressed mood; the overall effects may depend on the state of nicotine dependence and withdrawal.

Treatment of nicotine addiction

- Various *nicotine substitution* regimens available
  - These include gum, patches and inhalation.
  - E-cigarettes are closest in pharmacokinetic profile to smoking and their role as an alternative to cigarettes is a current topic of debate.
- *Amfebutamone (bupropion)* is a DA and probable NA reuptake inhibitor, which has been shown to aid smoking cessation.
- *Varenicline*
  - Nicotinic receptor partial agonist
  - Shown efficacy in trials for smoking cessation
  - Some initial concerns about treatment-emergent mood disturbance and suicidality (possibly an effect of treatment and/or smoking cessation) but can be used safely in psychiatric disorders
- *Rimonabant*: Cannabinoid CB_1 receptor antagonist, although showing some efficacy, has been withdrawn due to depression and suicidality as an adverse effect.

Marijuana

- Also known as cannabis, pot, weed, hash.
- *Main active chemical*: δ-9-tetrahydrocannabinol (THC) but up to 60 others, including cannabidiol which is antipsychotic. Concentration, and relative concentrations, of different active chemicals varies, which contributes to differences in psychological and adverse effects between preparations.
- Main effects of THC are mediated by binding to a G-protein-coupled receptor (the cannabinoid CB_1 receptor) leading to a reduction in cAMP and consequently neurotransmitter release.
- CB_1 receptors are located on the pre-synaptic terminal where they act to inhibit the release of classical neurotransmitters; they are not currently thought to be post-synaptic.
- Two putative endocannabinoid ligands for CB_1 receptor are arachidonylethanolamine (anandamide) and 2-arachidonylglycerol (2-AG).
- Anandamide has been proposed to function in a 'retrograde' manner. When a post-synaptic neuron is depolarised, anandamide is synthesised and released from the post-synaptic neuron to exert its effects through CB_1 receptors on the pre-synaptic neuron (see Chapter 1).
- Highest concentrations of CB_1 receptors are found in the basal ganglia and cerebellum (movement) and portions of the hippocampal formation (memory); moderately dense binding is found throughout the neocortex, particularly in the frontal, limbic and temporal lobes (cognitive and emotional functions).
- Cannabinoid CB_2 receptors are found on immune cells.
- A distinction needs to be made between smoked cannabis and cannabis-based medicines which are showing efficacy, for example cannabinoid CB_1 receptor agonists in appetite stimulation, spasticity and neuropathic pain and cannabinoid CB_1 receptor antagonists in smoking cessation and obesity (note that rimonabant has been withdrawn due to association with depression and suicide).
- Evidence from animal models supports a role for the cannabinoid system in mediating effects of other drugs such as opioids and alcohol. It may also be involved in mood regulation.

Effects of cannabis

- *Acute effects*: Relaxation, time confusion, feeling of 'well-being', distorted perceptions, impairment of memory, concentration and coordination, increased pulse, appetite, anxiety.
- *Chronic effects*: 'Amotivational syndrome' – impaired attention, memory, learning, drive.
- Dependence syndrome.

- *Psychotomimetic effects*: These do not occur with everyone and generally resolve.
- More controversial as to whether it causes enduring psychotic illness de novo. Evidence supports risk in precipitating and exacerbating psychosis, particularly in young people, and is associated with poorer prognosis in schizophrenia.
- Smoking associated with respiratory problems, lung cancer and cardiovascular disease.

Other drugs

γ-Hydroxybutyrate

- γ-Hydroxybutyrate (GHB) and its prodrugs gamma-butyrolactone (GBL) and 1,4-butanediol are central nervous system depressants; street names include 'GBH' and 'liquid ecstasy'.
- Its main effects are mediated through GHB and $GABA_B$ receptors.
- GHB can cause respiratory arrest, particularly with alcohol.
- GHB is used recreationally for its sedative, stimulant and pro-sexual effects (and has been used as a date-rape drug).

Benzodiazepines

These are discussed in Chapter 6.

Bibliography

Guidelines

Department of Health. Drug misuse and dependence: UK guidelines on clinical management. 2007; http://www.nta.nhs.uk/uploads/clinical_guidelines_2007.pdf.

Lingford-Hughes AR, Welch S, Peters L et al. BAP updated guidelines: Evidence-based guidelines for the pharmacological management of substance abuse, harmful use, addiction and comorbidity: Recommendations from BAP. *J Psychopharmacol.* 2012; 26: 899–952. http://www.bap.org.uk/pdfs/BAPaddictionEBG_2012.pdf.

National Institute for Health and Care Excellence. Drug misuse – opioid detoxification. *NICE Clinical Guideline 185.* 2007; http://www.nice.org.uk/guidance/cg52.

National Institute for Health and Care Excellence. Methadone and buprenorphine for the management of opioid dependence. NICE technology appraisal guidance 111. 2007; http://www.nice.org.uk/guidance/ta114.

National Institute for Health and Care Excellence. Naltrexone for the management of opioid dependence. *NICE Technology Appraisal Guidance 115.* 2007; http://www.nice.org.uk/guidance/ta115.

National Institute for Health and Care Excellence. Varenicline for smoking cessation. *NICE Technology Appraisal Guidance 123*. 2007; http://www.nice.org.uk/guidance/ta123.

National Institute for Health and Care Excellence. Smoking cessation services. *NICE Public Health Guidance 10*. 2008 (modified 2013); http://www.nice.org.uk/guidance/ph10 (section on pharmacotherapies for smoking cessation).

National Institute for Health and Care Excellence. Alcohol-use disorders: Diagnosis, assessment and management of harmful drinking and alcohol dependence. *NICE Clinical Guideline 115*. 2011; http://www.nice.org.uk/guidance/cg115.

National Institute for Health and Care Excellence. Nalmefene for reducing alcohol consumption in people with alcohol dependence. *NICE Technology Appraisal Guidance 325*. 2014; http://www.nice.org.uk/guidance/ta325.

Key references

Iversen L. Cannabis and the brain. *Brain*. 2003; 126: 1252–1270.

Koob GF, Volkow ND. Neurocircuitry of addiction. *Neuropsychopharmacology*. 2010; 35: 217–238.

Kreek MJ, LaForge KS, Butelman E. Pharmacotherapy of addictions. *Nat Rev Drug Discov*. 2002; 1: 710–726.

Lingford-Hughes A, Watson B, Kalk N, Reid A. Neuropharmacology of addiction and how it informs treatment. *Br Med Bull*. 2010; 96: 93–110.

Sellman D. The 10 most important things known about addiction. *Addiction*. 2010; 105: 6–13.

Further reading

Addiction is a brain disease, and it matters. A series of articles in *Science*. 1997; 278: 45–70.

European Monitoring Centre for Drugs and Drug Addiction. Synthetic cathinone drug profile, 2015; http://www.emcdda.europa.eu/publications/drug-profiles/synthetic-cathinones.

Farren CK, Hill KP, Weiss RD. Bipolar disorder and alcohol use disorder: A review. *Curr Psychiatry Rep*. 2012; 14: 659–666.

Green AI, Drake RE, Brunette MF, Noordsy DL. Schizophrenia and co-occurring substance use disorder. *Am J Psychiatry*. 2007; 164: 402–408.

Drugs for dementia and cognitive impairment

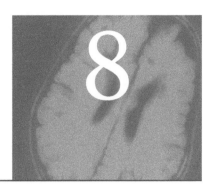

Mehran Javeed, Ian M Anderson and Iracema Leroi

 ## Introduction

The risk of developing dementia increases with age, occurring in one in six people over the age of 80 years. Alzheimer's disease (AD) is the most common dementia, making up about 60% of cases.

- Two main types of symptoms have been a focus of treatment in dementia and related disorders:
  - Cognitive deficits
  - Non-cognitive features (behavioural and psychological symptoms of dementia [BPSD], consisting of affective, psychotic and behavioural disturbances)

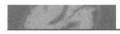 ## History

- Deficits in the acetylcholine (ACh) system in AD led to a focus on drug approaches to enhance ACh function:
  - Initial studies with ACh precursors did not show benefit.
  - *Acetylcholinesterase inhibitors (AChEIs)*: Tacrine introduced as a cognitive enhancer in AD in the 1980s and licensed for AD in 1993 (United States).
  - Second-generation AChEIs have improved adverse effect profiles.
- The NMDA receptor antagonist memantine, originally introduced to improve motor performance in Parkinson's disease (PD), is licensed for AD in the United States and European Union.
- Interest in other drugs to enhance cognition (nootropics), covering a wider range from phytochemicals (e.g. ginkgo biloba) to stimulant drugs, has not, as yet, provided clinically useful drugs.

Neurobiology of dementia

Alzheimer's disease

Neuropathology

- In AD there is initially localised loss of neurons especially in the hippo-campus and basal forebrain; the type and function of the neurons and pathways affected determine the clinical picture, such as the cognitive and memory deficits seen early in the disease.
- Two characteristic microscopic features are extracellular amyloid plaques consisting of β-*amyloid protein* (Aβ) and intraneuronal *neurofibrillary tangles* associated with phosphorylated Tau protein (see Figure 8.1 for a simplified scheme).

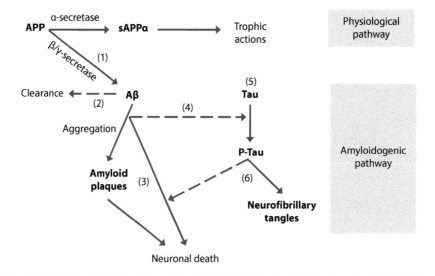

Figure 8.1 Simplified pathology of AD. Amyloid precursor protein (APP) is normally cleaved by α-secretase to form soluble APP alpha (sAPPα) which is involved in cell growth, synaptic formation and repair. Cleavage at different points by β- and γ-secretases (1) leads to the formation of β-amyloid (Aβ), a process favoured by APP and presenilin mutations (some cases of familial AD). Clearance of Aβ (2) is impaired by a polymorphism of the apolipoprotein E gene (ApoE ε4), involved in lipoprotein and cholesterol transport; ApoE ε4 is a risk factor for sporadic AD. Aβ aggregates to form oligopolymers and amyloid plaques (3), which lead to cell death by mechanisms including inflammation and increased vulnerability to ischaemia, excitotoxicity and oxidative stress. Tau (associated with intracellular microtubules) is hyperphosphorylated (P-Tau) in the presence of Aβ (4). P-Tau formation is also favoured by some Tau gene polymorphisms (5); P-Tau forms paired helical filaments which enhance Aβ neurotoxicity and also aggregate to form neurofibrillary tangles (6).

- The pathological pathway potentially offers multiple sites for therapeutic interventions, but at present only two systems (cholinergic and glutamatergic) are targeted by licensed drugs (see next sections).
- Risk factors for AD include ageing, mild cognitive impairment (MCI), genetic polymorphisms or mutations (Figure 8.1), family history of AD, female sex, lower educational level, head injury and type II diabetes.

Cholinergic neurotransmission

- Figure 8.2 outlines the main metabolic pathways of ACh (see also Chapter 1).
  - Central nervous system (CNS) cholinergic pathways are involved in attention and memory, perception, sleep and mood, and in the periphery it is a neurotransmitter in the parasympathetic nervous system and in innervation of skeletal muscle.
  - Antimuscarinic agents (e.g. scopolamine) can cause memory impairment and confusion.
- In AD there is substantial loss of cholinergic neurons in the *nucleus basalis of Meynert*, the origin of the cholinergic pathway projecting to cortical areas and thalamus:
  - Post-mortem estimates of cholinergic function correlate with mental test scores and amyloid plaque counts.
  - Choline acetyltransferase (ChAT), choline uptake and ACh release in the neocortex are reduced (Figure 8.2).

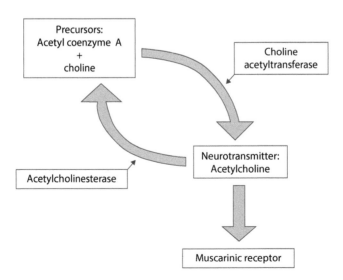

Figure 8.2 The metabolic pathway of ACh.

- Two cholinesterases are present in the body:
  - Acetylcholinesterase (AChE) found in cholinergic synapses in the CNS and periphery.
  - Butyrylcholinesterase (BuChE, previously known as pseudocholinesterase) synthesised in the liver and secreted into plasma; its inhibition may lead to unwanted peripheral side effects. It is also present in glial cells.

Glutamatergic neurotransmission

- Glutamate is the major excitatory neurotransmitter in the CNS (see Chapter 1); cortical and hippocampal pyramidal neurons are glutamatergic.
- Aß stimulates glutamatergic neurons which may lead to excitotoxic cell death by increasing the influx of Ca^{2+}.
- Prevention or reduction of this influx by blocking the glutamate NMDA receptor (e.g. by memantine) may be neuroprotective.

Monoaminergic neurotransmission

- *Noradrenaline (NA)*
  - Loss of locus coeruleus NA neurons may be associated with depressive symptoms and attentional deficits.
  - Relative preservation/slightly elevated levels of substantia nigra NA have been associated with delusions.
- *Serotonin (5-HT)*
  - Loss of 5-HT neurons is most prominent in the temporal cortex, hippocampus and amygdala.
  - Impaired 5-HT function may be associated with aggression, depression and other aspects of BPSD.
- *Dopamine (DA)*
  - DA and L-DOPA are reduced in mesolimbic and mesocortical areas in AD.
  - Aß oligomers impair DA release.
  - DA receptor and COMT polymorphisms have been associated with behavioural dyscontrol and psychosis.

Other mechanisms

The neuropathology of AD involves many other processes potentially amenable to prevention and/or treatment including the following:

- The amyloid pathway
- Tau phosphorylation

- Inflammation/immune pathways
- Oxidation and free radicals
- Neurotoxic processes including Ca^{2+} influx
- Systemic factors involved in cerebrovascular disease

Other dementias and mild cognitive impairment

- *Vascular dementia* (VaD)
    - For example, multi-infarct dementia, small vessel dementia and infarcts of strategic areas.
    - Vascular risk factors, such as diabetes, high cholesterol and lipids and hypertension, are major contributing factors.
    - AD and VaD share many risk factors and it has been proposed that their pathologies are overlapping, for example, in inflammatory/immune pathways.
- *Dementia with Lewy bodies* (DLB) and *Parkinson's disease dementia* (PDD)
    - Are characterised by the presence of intraneuronal Lewy bodies (aggregations of alpha-synuclein, a protein believed to be involved in synaptic vesicle function) which lead to cell death.
    - Hippocampal atrophy is relatively mild.
    - Cholinergic and nigrostriatal DAergic systems are among those impaired (the latter causing exquisite sensitivity to DA blockade by antipsychotics).
    - The core features of DLB are fluctuating cognitive impairment, vivid visual hallucinations and Parkinsonian symptoms.
    - Dementia in PDD occurs much later in the illness than occurs in DLB, but it appears to share the same underlying pathology.
- *Frontotemporal dementia*
    - Is predominantly an early-onset dementia (previously called Pick's disease) with clinical symptoms reflecting the location of neuronal loss (personality and behaviour change, blunting of emotions and language deficits).
    - Familial and genetic factors are more common than other dementias, including mutations in Tau genes.
- *Mild cognitive impairment* (MCI)
    - Is defined as concern about, and impairment of, cognition (one or more domains) in the absence of dementia and with continued independence. Only a minority (<5%–20%) progress to dementia.
    - Is a syndromal diagnosis and has no single specific pathology, with many of the same risk factors as for AD.

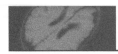

Assessment of outcome in drug trials for dementia

- Assessment is difficult, involving a number of domains (Table 8.1).
- Interpretation can be problematic; prevention of deterioration is as important as improvement, requiring trials of sufficient duration.
- There is increasing need to recognise the 'minimum clinically important difference' which patient or carer thinks is sufficient for a change in management, as well as patient-reported outcome measures (PROMs).
- Evidence is greatest for AD, with limited data for other types of dementia.
- The BAP guidelines (see Guidelines) on anti-dementia drugs have a brief discussion about some methodological issues in clinical trials in dementia.

Table 8.1 Assessment domains and main associated rating scales in drug trials for dementia

Cognitive performance/function
Alzheimer's Disease Assessment Scale (ADAS-cog): Tests multiple areas of cognitive decline.
Mini Mental State Examination (MMSE): Screening instrument briefly tests several areas of cognition but not in depth.
Numerous others available

Global outcome measures
Clinicians' Interview-Based Impression of Change (CIBIC): Interview-based assessment of global functioning. CIBIC-plus includes interview with carer. Usually, a primary outcome variable.
Clinical Dementia Rating (CDR): Six domains rating deterioration in ability.

Functional ability/activities of daily living (ADL)
Instrumental Activities of Daily Living (IADL): Assesses ability on household tasks.
Interview for Deterioration in Daily living in Dementia (IDDD): Assesses deterioration in simple and more complex areas of daily living activity.

Behaviour and mood
Neuropsychiatric Inventory (NPI): Assesses psychiatric and behavioural changes in 12 domains.
Behavioural Pathology in Alzheimer's Disease scale (BEHAVE-AD): Clinician interview of behavioural domains, including psychotic and affective symptoms.
Cornell Scale for Depression in Dementia

Drugs for cognitive impairment

- Table 8.2 lists the drugs currently licensed for the treatment of cognitive impairment in dementia.
- There is limited evidence for drug treatment for the prevention of dementia and for treatments modifying illness progression. Some long-term observational studies suggest that treatment with AChEIs and memantine in AD may be associated with slower decline in cognition and function.

Table 8.2 Drugs licensed for the treatment of cognitive impairment in dementia

Drug	Mechanism of action	Metabolism	Elimination half-life	Preparations	Adverse effect and interactions
Donepezil	Selective reversible AChE inhibitor	CYP 2D6, CYP 3A4	70–80 h	Tablets/ orodis-persible tablets	GI side effects are dose related. Rarer adverse effects are stomach ulcers, sinoatrial block and atrio-ventricular block, seizures and transient ischaemic attacks. Caution with concomitant CYP inducers and inhibitors
Galantamine	Reversible AChE inhibitor, presynaptic nAChR modulator	CYP 2D6, CYP 3A4	8–10 h, but slow release available	Tablets/ capsules/ oral solution	
Rivastigmine	Pseudo-irreversible AChE and BuChE inhibitor	Minimal hepatic involvement	Less than 2 h	Capsules/ oral solution/ patches	
Memantine	Low affinity, non-competitive NMDA receptor antagonist	Minimal hepatic involvement	60–80 h	Tablets/oral drops	Can cause hallucinations and worsen confusion. Levels increased with ranitidine and cimetidine.

Notes: AChE, acetylcholinesterase; AChR, acetylcholine receptor; BuChE, butyrylcholinesterase; CYP, cytochrome; NMDA, N-methyl-D-aspartate.

Cholinergic drugs

- *Cholinergic precursors* (choline and lecithin, a dietary source of choline), and an ACh releaser (linopirdine), have not been not found to be effective in AD.
- *Cholinergic agonists* have shown lack of evidence and/or poor tolerability in clinical trials.

Acetylcholinesterase inhibitors

- The actions of AChEIs depend on intact cholinergic nerve terminals and therefore their effects are lost with disease progression.
- Details of the three licensed AChEI, *donepezil, galantamine and rivastigmine*, are given in Table 8.2.
- *Clinical evidence*
  - Meta-analyses of randomised controlled trials (RCTs) in AD show that all three drugs are effective for cognitive, global and functional domains; behavioural benefit is most established for galantamine, but has not been shown for rivastigmine. Evidence is lacking for preventing institutionalisation (although a trend for donepezil has been reported).
  - The modest benefits on cognitive function appear independent of the degree of cognitive impairment.
  - They are cost-effective in comparison with best supportive care.
  - They also appear effective for LBD and PDD.
  - There is limited evidence suggesting possible benefit in cognitive and global domains in VaD.
  - They are not effective for MCI but cause GI adverse effects.
- *Metrifonate* (not licensed, currently unavailable)
  - Originally developed to treat schistosomiasis.
  - First AChEI with established efficacy for AD from RCTs; a meta-analysis found efficacy in global, cognitive and functional domains.
  - Generally well tolerated, side effects mainly GI and muscle weakness.
- *Tacrine (tetrahydroaminoacridine)*
  - First licensed AChEI for AD (United States) but licence withdrawn in 2013 given safer alternative drugs (it is associated with hepatotoxicity and requirement for LFT monitoring).
  - Meta-analysis of RCTs shows efficacy in cognitive and global domains in AD, but functional benefit is uncertain.
- Other AChEIs in AD
  - *Huperzine A* (a reversible AChEI derived from the Chinese herb *Huperzia serrata*) first identified in the 1980s: A meta-analysis suggested benefit on cognitive, functional and global domains, but trial quality is poor.

- *Physostigmine* (a reversible AChEI occurring naturally in the Calabar bean): Showed preliminary evidence for efficacy but is poorly tolerated.
- *Phenserine* (a non-competitive AChEI with modulatory effects on Aβ generation): Has preliminary evidence for efficacy.
- *Ladostigil* (inhibitor of AChEI and BuChE and a brain-selective MAOI): Currently in early clinical trials.

Glutamatergic drugs

Memantine

- The only licensed glutamatergic drug for AD. See Table 8.2 for details.
- Antagonism of NMDA receptors is believed to underlie its efficacy in AD.
- It is also a non-competitive antagonist at 5-HT_3 and nicotinic ACh receptors and an agonist at D_2 receptors. Their contribution to its clinical effects is unknown.
- *Clinical evidence*
  - Meta-analyses of RCTs in AD show efficacy in global and functional domains and trends to benefit in cognition and behaviour.
  - Functional benefit is greater in more severe illness.
  - Efficacy appears comparable to donepezil.
  - It is used in combination with AChEIs; however, the combination has not been shown to add benefit compared with monotherapy.
  - Cost-effectiveness is less well established than for AChEIs.
  - Probably little role in VaD; some evidence for cognitive, but not global, benefit.
  - Results are inconsistent in a few small studies in DLB and PDD; a meta-analysis suggested a modest global benefit in PDD.

Other glutamatergic drugs

- There have been relatively few trials of other glutamatergic drugs with conflicting open evidence for D-cycloserine (partial agonist at glycine site of NMDA receptor) and lack of efficacy in an RCT of an AMPA potentiator.

Drugs acting on other systems

Although there are numerous potential targets, based on the pathology of the AD (Figure 8.1) and other dementias, no treatments based on these have established clinical benefit.

- *Amyloid pathway*
  - In spite of considerable interest and investigation, to date treatments modifying the amyloid pathway have shown no benefit, and sometimes harm.
  - Ineffective approaches have included active and passive immunisation against Aß, ß/γ-secretase inhibitors, increasing Aß clearance with rosiglitazone and attenuating Aß oligomerisation with metal protein attenuating compounds (MPACs).
- *Tau protein*: Glycogen synthase kinase-3 (GSK-3) is an enzyme responsible for tau phosphorylation, and inhibitors (which include methylene blue) are currently in phase II and III trials in AD.
- *Antioxidants* are hypothesised to prevent the neurotoxic effects of Aß, or the consequences of cerebrovascular disease; however, limited RCT evidence has not found a benefit from antioxidants such as vitamin E in AD or MCI. Epidemiological studies of antioxidant intake (including coffee) have provided conflicting data on whether or not they can reduce the risk of dementia.
- *Inflammation/immunotherapy*
  - RCTs of steroidal and non-steroidal anti-inflammatory drugs (NSAIDs) have not been found to benefit patients with established AD; instead there is a trend to higher death rates with NSAIDs, especially with selective cyclooxygenase-2 (COX-2) inhibitors.
  - Epidemiological studies have suggested that NSAIDs might delay the onset of AD, all-cause dementia and MCI.
  - Propentofylline (a xanthine derivative which inhibits adenosine reuptake and phosphodiesterase) is believed to modify immune processes but has shown limited benefit in cognition, global function and function in AD or VaD.
- *Other agents*
  - Systematic reviews have found that antihypertensives lower the risk of developing VaD and the progression of symptoms.
  - Statins may have a slight protective effect against the onset of AD or VaD in observational studies, but confounding factors are likely to explain this.
  - A meta-analysis of poor-quality RCTs of naftidrofuryl, a vasodilator, found no global effect in dementia, although some benefits on performance, behaviour, cognition and mood were found; it was well tolerated.
  - A meta-analysis of RCTs of selegiline (a MAOI-B inhibitor) found improvement in short-term cognition and function in AD, but this was not sustained beyond 8 weeks.
  - A meta-analysis of nimodipine, a Ca^{2+} channel blocker, found short-term benefit on global, cognitive and general psychopathology scales, but not function, in AD, VaD and mixed dementia.

- A systematic review of natural medicines found that ginkgo biloba may have a small effect on cognition and function in AD, but did not appear to reduce the risk of its occurrence.
- Evidence from epidemiological studies suggests that omega-3 fatty acids may reduce the risk of AD and MCI, but a systematic review of RCTs found that it was ineffective in treating AD. A small benefit was found in MCI for attention and processing speed, but not for memory or executive function.
- There is no evidence that oestrogen hormone replacement therapy (HRT) in women reduces the risk of dementia.

 # Behavioural and psychological symptoms of dementia (BPSD)

- BPSD refers to non-cognitive symptoms seen in individuals with dementia.
- Up to 90% of people with dementia will develop BPSD at some point in their illness, which can result in an increase in caregiver burden.
- The presence of BPSD may also precipitate institutionalisation, which is associated with an increased cost of care.

Drug treatments for BPSD

- Given the constellation of symptoms of mood, behaviour and disturbed perception, successful management of BPSD requires awareness that causes are often multifactorial.
- No drugs apart from risperidone (see Antipsychotics section) are licensed for BPSD.
- Table 8.3 outlines a pharmacological approach to specific target symptoms in BPSD.

Antipsychotics

- Antipsychotics have been used in dementia care for decades but have been controversial.
- The development and use of atypical antipsychotics brought to light an increased risk of cerebrovascular-related events in dementia. A three fold increase risk of stroke was found with risperidone and olanzapine compared to placebo; this increased risk is now thought to apply to all antipsychotics.
- RCTs have established that olanzapine and risperidone are effective for aggression and psychosis in AD. Risperidone is the only drug licensed

Table 8.3   Pharmacological approaches to target symptoms in BPSD

Target symptom	Drug treatment
Depression	SSRIs and mirtazapine: Poor evidence for clinical efficacy. SSRIs fairly well tolerated but risk of GI bleeding, especially with aspirin or NSAIDs. TCAs: Poor evidence for efficacy and avoid due to cholinergic side effects.
Psychosis	Risperidone: Effective in managing psychotic symptoms with less evidence to support other atypical antipsychotics; caution due to increased risk of mortality and stroke. Antidepressants: No significant benefit. AChEIs: Show some benefit. Rivastigmine: Improvement in hallucinations in DLB.
Agitation	Risperidone: Effective in managing agitation. Memantine: Modest evidence for efficacy. Trazodone, carbamazepine, valproate: Very limited evidence of clinical benefit. Benzodiazepines: No evidence for significant benefit; caution due to increased risk of falls and worsening cognition.
Apathy	AChEIs: Modestly effective in managing apathy. Methylphenidate: Limited evidence of benefit; caution due to side effects such as anxiety and weight loss.
Insomnia	Trazodone: May improve total sleep time and sleep efficiency. No benefit from melatonin or ramelteon. There is a lack of evidence for common clinically used drugs (e.g. antihistamines, benzodiazepines and antipsychotics).
Sexual disinhibition	SSRIs: May reduce libido and cause sexual dysfunction and appear first line. TCAs: May reduce libido but can worsen cognition. Antipsychotics: DA antagonism and antimuscarinic properties may reduce libido and arousal; this may be especially in prolactin-elevating drugs such as haloperidol and risperidone. Caution with mirtazapine and benzodiazepines which can both cause hypersexuality. Antiandrogens: Limited evidence with agents such as medroxyprogesterone acetate and cyproterone acetate; caution as they can cause hypotension and liver damage.

for short-term treatment of persistent aggression in AD in the European Union/United Kingdom, with none licensed in the United States.

- Quetiapine, clozapine and olanzapine have some evidence for efficacy in treating psychotic symptoms in DLB.
- The emphasis now is to closely monitor and minimise the use of anti-psychotics in dementia (e.g. the 2009 National Dementia Strategy for England).

Antidepressants

- The most recent meta-analyses have found SSRIs ineffective in treating depression or cognition in AD, although they may be helpful for agitation.
- Evidence is extremely limited for other antidepressants, with inconclusive studies for TCAs in treating depression in AD.

Acetylcholinesterase inhibitors and memantine

- AChEIs only have a small effect on BPSD in AD which is of uncertain clinical importance.
- In DLB, psychotic symptoms – particularly visual hallucinations – appear to respond well to AChEIs.
- Memantine may have some efficacy in reducing agitation.

Treatment of cognitive impairment in other disorders

- Cognitive impairment also occurs in non-degenerative conditions such as schizophrenia, bipolar disorder and depression and as a result of head trauma.
- Potentially there are risks and neuropathological (e.g. inflammatory) factors shared with degenerative disorders such as AD.
- *Later-life depression* is often associated with more cognitive deficits, particularly executive dysfunction, than depression in younger individuals; depression is also a risk factor for, or prodrome of, dementia. Cognition improves with treatment of depression, and evidence is lacking for benefits from cognitive enhancers.
- In *schizophrenia/schizoaffective disorder*
  - Adjunctive AChEI may have some benefit on negative and overall psychiatric symptoms, but do not improve cognition.
  - Modafinil may improve negative symptoms, but, although some single dose trials showed improvement in attentional set-shifting and verbal memory, treatment trials have not shown cognitive benefit.

- Hopes that atypical antipsychotics might improve cognitive function (e.g. by effects at 5-HT receptor subtypes such as 5-HT_{1A}, 5-HT_6 or 5-HT_7 receptors) have not to date been realised.
- Cognitive impairment is seen in euthymic patients with *bipolar disorder*. Attempting to minimise cognitive adverse effects from lithium and anticonvulsants is important, but the effect of cognitive enhancers has been little studied.
- *Traumatic brain injury* can cause cognitive impairment and slightly increases the risk of dementia. AChEIs modestly improve memory and attention.

Principles of prescribing for dementia

- The general principles for prescribing to a mainly elderly population apply (see Chapter 11).
- Non-pharmacological approaches are the mainstay for managing dementia and reduce the need for symptomatic medication; key to these are a suitable environment and a patient-centred approach with adequate support for carers and sufficient time, numbers and training of staff:
  - Specific strategies for cognitive impairment/maintaining cognitive function include structured group stimulation, memory aids, cognitive training and cognitive rehabilitation.
  - For BPSD, options include multisensory stimulation, music and dance, aromatherapy, animal therapy, reminiscence therapy and massage.
- In the United Kingdom, for the pharmacological treatment of cognitive impairment, NICE guidance recommends the following:
  - The three licensed AChEIs as an option for mild-to-moderate AD.
  - Memantine as an option for moderate AD, if AChEIs are contraindicated or not tolerated, and for severe AD.
  - That AChEIs are not used for VaD or MCI unless part of a clinical trial.
  - Treatment should be initiated by specialists in dementia care; involve regular cognitive, global, functional and behavioural assessment; and continued only as long as it is beneficial.
- For pharmacological treatment of BPSD, NICE guidance recommends the following:
  - That antipsychotics should only be used for severe symptoms in dementia, after a careful assessment of risks and benefits for individual drugs; initial doses should be low and treatment time limited, with careful monitoring of target symptoms and adverse effects.
  - AChEIs as an option for mild-to-moderate dementias (apart from VaD) after failure of non-drug measures or antipsychotics, with memantine a subsequent option.

- In contrast to NICE, other European guidelines emphasise the early use of AChEI in dementia, as well as wider indications for memantine. The BAP guidelines on anti-dementia drugs give a useful review of the evidence and evidence-based consensus guidance for the different dementias.

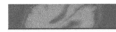 ## Acknowledgement

This is an update and revision of the third edition chapter by Harry Allen.

 ## Bibliography

Guidelines

National Institute for Health and Care Excellence. Donepezil, galantamine, rivastigmine and memantine for the treatment of Alzheimer's disease. *NICE Technology Appraisal Guidance 217.* 2011; http://www.nice.org.uk/guidance/ta217.

National Institute for Health and Care Excellence. Dementia: Supporting people with dementia and their carers in health and social care. *NICE Clinical Guideline 42.* 2011; http://www.nice.org.uk/guidance/cg42.

O'Brien JT, Burns A, BAP Dementia Consensus Group. Clinical practice with anti-dementia drugs: A revised (second) consensus statement from the British Association for Psychopharmacology. *J Psychopharm.* 2010; 25: 997–1019. http://bap.org.uk/pdfs/Anti-dementia_2010_BAP.pdf.

Waldermar G, Dubois B, Emre M et al. Recommendations for the diagnosis and management of Alzheimer's disease and other disorders associated with dementia: EFNS guideline. *Eur J Neurol.* 2007; 14: e1–e26.

Key references

Aarsland D, Ballard C, Rongve A et al. Clinical trials of dementia with Lewy bodies and Parkinson's disease dementia. *Curr Neurol Neurosci Rep.* 2012; 12: 492–501.

Ballard CG, Waite J, Birks J. Atypical antipsychotics for aggression and psychosis in Alzheimer's disease. *Cochrane Database Syst Rev.* 2006; 1: CD003476.

Choi KH, Wykes T, Kurtz MM. Adjunctive pharmacotherapy for cognitive deficits in schizophrenia: Meta-analytical investigation of efficacy. *Br J Psychiatry.* 2013; 203: 172–178.

Di Santo SG, Prinelli F, Adorni F et al. A meta-analysis of the efficacy of donepezil, rivastigmine, galantamine, and memantine in relation to severity of Alzheimer's disease. *J Alzheimers Dis.* 2013; 35: 349–361.

Jaturapatporn D, Isaac MG, McCleery J, Tabet N. Aspirin, steroidal and non-steroidal anti-inflammatory drugs for the treatment of Alzheimer's disease. *Cochrane Database Syst Rev.* 2012; 2: CD006378.

Rolinski M, Fox C, Maidment I, McShane R. Cholinesterase inhibitors for dementia with Lewy bodies, Parkinson's disease dementia and cognitive impairment in Parkinson's disease. *Cochrane Database Syst Rev.* 2012; 3: CD006504.

Russ TC, Morling JR. Cholinesterase inhibitors for mild cognitive impairment. *Cochrane Database Syst Rev.* 2012; 9: CD009132.

Saddichha S, Pandey V. Alzheimer's and non-Alzheimer's dementia: A critical review of pharmacological and nonpharmacological strategies. *Am J Alzheimers Dis Other Demen.* 2008; 23: 150–161.

Sepehry AA, Lee PE, Hsiung GY et al. Effect of selective serotonin reuptake inhibitors in Alzheimer's disease with comorbid depression: A meta-analysis of depression and cognitive outcomes. *Drugs Aging.* 2012; 29: 793–806.

Shah K, Qureshi SU, Johnson M et al. Does use of antihypertensive drugs affect the incidence or progression of dementia? A systematic review. *Am J Geriatr Pharmacother.* 2009; 7: 250–261.

Tucker I. Management of inappropriate sexual behaviours in dementia: A literature review. *Int Psychogeriatr.* 2010; 22: 683–692.

Wong WB, Lin VW, Boudreau D, Devine EB. Statins in the prevention of dementia and Alzheimer's disease: A meta-analysis of observational studies and an assessment of confounding. *Pharmacoepidemiol Drug Saf.* 2013; 22: 345–358.

Further reading

Banerjee S, Hellier J, Dewey M et al. Sertraline or mirtazapine for depression in dementia (HTA-SADD): A randomised, multicentre, double-blind, placebo-controlled trial. *Lancet.* 2011; 378(9789): 403–411.

Birks J, López-Arrieta J. Nimodipine for primary degenerative, mixed and vascular dementia. *Cochrane Database Syst Rev.* 2002; 3: CD000147.

McKeith I, Dickson D, Emre M et al. Dementia with Lewy Bodies: Diagnosis and management: Third report of the DLB consortium. *Neurology.* 2005; 65: 1863–1872.

Mitchell AJ, Shiri-Feshki M. Rate of progression of mild cognitive impairment to dementia – Meta-analysis of 41 robust inception cohort studies. *Acta Psychiatr Scand.* 2009; 119: 252–265.

Tampi RR, Tampi DJ. Efficacy and tolerability of benzodiazepines for the treatment of behavioral and psychological symptoms of dementia: A systematic review of randomized controlled trials. *Am J Alzheimers Dis Other Demen.* 2014; 29: 565–574.

van de Glind EMM, van Enst WA, van Munster BC et al. Pharmacological treatment of dementia: A scoping review of systematic reviews. *Dement Geriatr Cogn Disord.* 2013; 36: 211–228.

Yi-Chun Y, Wen-Chen O. Mood stabilizers for the treatment of behavioral and psychological symptoms of dementia: An update review. *Kaohsiung J Med Sci.* 2012; 28: 185–193.

Drugs used for personality disorders and behavioural disturbance

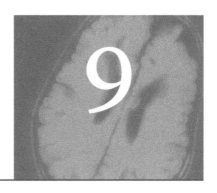

Birgit A Völlm and Ian M Anderson

- This chapter combines two rather disparate clinical issues – the pharmacological treatment of personality disorders and rapid tranquillisation (RT).
- The two topics do, however, have factors in common, namely.
  - Pharmacotherapy is targeted principally at symptoms and behaviour rather than directly at an underlying disorder.
  - Drug treatment is only indicated after psychosocial approaches have not worked, or cannot be used.
  - Careful consideration of risks and benefits in individual situations is required.
  - There is a lack of high-quality evidence.

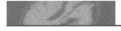 ## Drug treatment for personality disorders

Background

- The pharmacological treatment of personality disorders is relatively poorly researched and evidenced.
- Clinical trials to date have, in general, studied few patients, had short durations of treatment (weeks), tended to use inconsistent outcome measures and had high dropout rates.
- Despite the limited evidence, many patients with borderline personality disorder are prescribed medication, often more than one drug.
- There has been an increase in research recently, though mostly focussed on female outpatients with borderline personality disorder and low illness severity.
- Recent Cochrane reviews have summarised the evidence for borderline personality disorder and antisocial personality disorder (ASPD) but no systematic reviews currently exist for any of the other personality disorders.

Classification of personality disorder

- The *DSM-IV* classification system has been the most widely used classification system in clinical research with personality disordered subjects. In *DSM-5* the diagnostic criteria have not changed in the main manual, but the distinction between personality disorders and other mental disorders has been removed.
- In order to receive the diagnosis, individuals have to fulfil general criteria for personality disorder as well as specific criteria for each of the 10 different personality disorder types.
- Disorders are grouped into three clusters (A, B and C; see Table 9.1).

Table 9.1 Diagnostic criteria and types of personality disorder (based on *DSM-IV/5*)

Diagnosis
   General criteria for personality disorder
      An enduring pattern of inner experience and behaviour that deviates markedly from the expectations of the individual's culture with abnormalities in at least two of the following areas: Cognition, affectivity (emotional responsivity), interpersonal functioning, impulse control.
      The pattern is inflexible and pervasive, stable and of long duration starting in adolescence or early adulthood and leads to clinically significant distress or impairment in functioning.
      Not better accounted for by another mental or physical disorder or the physiological effects of a substance.
Types
   Cluster A: Odd–eccentric personality disorders
      Paranoid
      Schizoid
      Schizotypal
   Cluster B: Dramatic–emotional–erratic personality disorders
      Antisocial
      Borderline
      Histrionic
      Narcissistic
   Cluster C: Anxious–fearful personality disorders
      Avoidant
      Dependent
      Obsessive compulsive

▨ There are significant problems with the classification system which has hindered clinical and basic research:
  - The diagnostic categories have overlapping features, and individuals are commonly comorbid for more than one personality disorder and comorbidity with other mental disorders is also common.
  - These two factors mean that clinical trials, even when utilising carefully applied diagnostic criteria, necessarily study heterogeneous populations of patients.
  - Persistence as a core definition of personality disorder has been challenged. A recent long-term follow-up study found that outcome in borderline personality disorder is far better than previously realised.
▨ A number of researchers have argued that personality pathology is best conceptualised using a dimensional rather than a categorical approach. Proposals along these lines were not accepted for the recent *DSM-5* revision, but an alternative hybrid dimensional–categorical model has been included in Section III of *DSM-5* in order to encourage further research.

Theoretical issues

▨ The aetiology of personality disorders is complex, encompassing genetic, biological and environmental/social factors.
▨ For example, in borderline personality disorder
  - The estimated monozygotic to dizygotic concordance ratio is as high as 5:1 in some twin studies (i.e. similar in magnitude to schizophrenia).
  - Recent neuroimaging studies suggest functional and structural changes in areas involved in the processing of emotions and stress in the frontal and temporal lobes.
  - There is a clear association with early childhood trauma.
▨ Attempts have been made to link dimensions of normal and abnormal personality to specific neurotransmitter systems in order to provide a rationale for pharmacotherapy. Cloninger and colleagues proposed a psychobiology of temperament (inherited tendencies) and character (environmentally acquired personality features) which relates
  - *Novelty seeking* (inherited tendency to exploratory activity and intense excitement in response to novel stimuli) to DA function
  - *Harm avoidance* (inherited tendency to respond intensely to aversive stimuli and to avoid punishment, novelty and non-reward) to 5-HT function
  - *Reward dependence* (inherited tendency to respond intensely to reward and maintenance of rewarded behaviour) to NA function

- Unfortunately, this neat notion has limited empirical support. It has, nonetheless, provided a useful framework and stimulus for research and a spur to thinking about personality disorder beyond a purely descriptive classification.
- Pharmacotherapy of personality disordered individuals can be thought of as based on three main rationales:
  - A presumed *illness spectrum* with an equivalent mental disorder (e.g. antipsychotics for paranoid personality disorder–schizophrenia spectrum; anxiolytics and SSRIs for avoidant personality disorder–anxiety disorder spectrum).
  - *Symptom relief*, rather than treatment of the core disorder. It is notable, for example, that in some studies of borderline personality disorder, antipsychotics may have beneficial effects which extend beyond 'psychosis-like symptoms' to impact on mood and self-harm.
  - *Theoretical grounds* (e.g. treatment of presumed low 5-HT conditions such as aggression/impulsivity/suicidality with SSRIs, based on putative neurochemistry of Cloninger's temperamental types).

Psychological treatment of personality disorders

- Psychological approaches provide the mainstay for the treatment of personality disorder.
- Systematic reviews emphasise the use of specific forms of psychotherapy for borderline personality disorder with dialectical behaviour therapy having the best evidence base. RCTs also support the use of mentalisation-based treatment, transference-focused therapy and interpersonal therapy, and the evidence base for the efficacy of such treatments is growing.
- For ASPD, approaches based on cognitive behavioural therapy (CBT) have the best evidence base.

Pharmacological treatment of borderline personality disorder (see Table 9.2)

- NICE guidelines do not currently support the use of pharmacotherapy for borderline personality disorder or its symptoms, except for the short-term (up to 1 week) use of sedatives (antihistamines) in crisis.
- Other guidelines and systematic reviews identify some evidence for the use of pharmacotherapy (see Table 9.2).
- The evidence base has been growing, with larger, higher quality, RCTs being initiated with lower dropout rates and improved diagnostic fidelity.

Table 9.2 Drugs with RCT evidence for use in personality disorders

Disorder/target symptoms	Drug
Schizotypal personality disorder	
Overall symptom severity, positive and negative symptoms	Risperidone[a]
Overall schizotypal personality symptoms	Risperidone
Borderline personality disorder	
Overall symptom severity	Quetiapine[b]
Interpersonal problems	Haloperidol
	Topiramate
	Valproate
Impulsivity	Lamotrigine
	Topiramate
	Valproate
Suicidal/self-harming behaviour	Flupentixol decanoate
	Omega-3 fatty acids
Affective instability	Aripiprazole
	Fluvoxamine
	Lamotrigine
	Olanzapine[c]
	Valproate
Intense anger	Aripiprazole
	Haloperidol
	Lamotrigine
	Olanzapine[c]
	Topiramate
	Valproate
Transient psychotic symptoms[a]	Aripiprazole
	Olanzapine[c]
	Topiramate
Antisocial personality disorder	
Impulsive aggression	Phenytoin
Avoidant personality disorder	
Overall symptom severity	Moclobemide[d]

No RCT evidence currently exists for the effectiveness of pharmacotherapy for the symptoms of fear of abandonment, identity disturbance or feelings of emptiness.

[a] Low dose up to 2 mg/day.
[b] Lower doses seem more beneficial than moderate ones.
[c] May increase suicidal ideation and self-harming behaviours.
[d] Comorbid social phobia, only high dose effective.

However, there remains a lack of consensus on outcome measures and an over reliance on subscale analysis.

- Most drug treatments do not influence total borderline personality disorder severity, nor change some core symptoms (chronic feelings of emptiness, identify disturbance, dissociation and avoidance of abandonment).
- However, certain drugs have been shown to positively affect other target symptoms.
- Pharmacological approaches mainly centre on three main classes of drugs: Antipsychotics, antidepressants and 'mood stabilisers', with different drug classes showing promise for different symptom profiles.

Antipsychotics (see Chapter 3)

- RCTs against placebo are available for first-generation antipsychotics (haloperidol, flupentixol decanoate, loxapine and thiothixene) and second-generation antipsychotics (aripiprazole, olanzapine, quetiapine and ziprasidone).
- Except for olanzapine and quetiapine, all treatment effect estimates are based on single RCTs.
  - *Haloperidol* has been shown to have a positive effect on anger and interpersonal problems but not on impulsivity and psychotic symptoms.
  - *Flupentixol decanoate* may reduce self-mutilating behaviours.
  - *Aripiprazole* may be effective in reducing symptoms of anger, impulsivity, self-mutilating behaviours, interpersonal problems and psychotic symptoms.
  - *Olanzapine* may reduce anger, affective instability and psychotic symptoms but not impulsivity; however, it may also increase suicidal ideation and self-harming behaviours compared to placebo.
  - *Quetiapine* may reduce overall symptom severity and disability with lower doses being more beneficial than moderate ones.
  - *Clozapine* may be beneficial in severe borderline personality disorder, including controlling psychotic symptoms, affective instability and self-harm, but evidence is only from case reports and small open-label studies.
  - Some antipsychotics appear to positively affect general and associated psychopathology such as depression and anxiety.

Antidepressants (see Chapter 4)

- TCAs (amitriptyline), MAOIs inhibitors (phenelzine) and SSRIs (fluoxetine and fluvoxamine) have all been evaluated in RCTs, but the evidence for their efficacy has been disappointing.

- No benefit has been found in any of these trials for symptoms of anger, impulsivity, suicidal ideation, self-harming behaviours, interpersonal problems or psychosis.
- One trial found an improvement in affective instability with fluvoxamine.
- Amitriptyline, but not SSRIs, has been shown to reduce depressive symptoms.

'Mood stabilisers' (see Chapter 5)

- Open-label studies exist for lithium and phenytoin, but due to their side effect profile, these drugs should be used with extreme caution in borderline personality disorder.
- The following significant effects have been found in RCTs:
  - *Valproate* has been helpful in the reduction of anger, impulsivity, affective instability and interpersonal problems but not for impulsivity or suicidal ideation.
  - *Lamotrigine* has shown a positive effect on symptoms of anger, impulsivity and affective instability.
  - *Topiramate* has shown a reduction in anger, impulsivity, interpersonal problems and psychotic symptoms.
  - *Carbamazepine* has shown no significant benefit in well-controlled trials.

Other agents

- BDZs are often used (or end up being used for a variety of reasons, including 'self-prescription') in patients with personality disorder. However
  - There is no substantial evidence that this class of drugs is of value, and there is a theoretical risk of disinhibition.
  - The risk of dependence may be greater in these patients.
  - Therefore, the usual considerations apply: Limit dose and length of use, and monitor for tolerance and dose escalation (see Chapter 6).
- Recently some RCT evidence has demonstrated effectiveness of omega-3 fatty acids in the reduction of suicidality and depressive symptoms.

Pharmacological treatment of antisocial personality disorder (see Table 9.2)

- NICE guidelines do not currently support the use of pharmacotherapy for ASPD or its symptoms.
- A Cochrane review has reported some evidence for the use of phenytoin, based on an RCT, in reducing the frequency and intensity of aggression in male prisoners.

- Historically lithium and carbamazepine have been used to reduce impulsivity and aggression, but good evidence for efficacy is lacking.
- In patients with ASPD and alcohol dependency, limited RCT evidence suggests an effect of nortriptyline and bromocriptine on anxiety.

Pharmacological treatment of other personality disorders (see Table 9.2)

- The evidence for the use of pharmacotherapy in other personality disorders is even more limited, and no guidelines currently exist.
- One RCT of risperidone showed reductions in positive and negative symptoms, as well as overall symptom severity, in schizotypal personality disorder but another study found no effect.
- Some studies have demonstrated effectiveness of antipsychotics in reducing conversion to schizophrenia in those with 'at risk mental states' which may include symptoms of schizotypal personality disorder.
- One large RCT of individuals with avoidant personality disorder, co-morbid with social phobia, showed a positive effect of high, compared to low, dose moclobemide on overall improvement.

Principles of drug therapy for personality disorder

Consider the following factors based on principles of good clinical practice:

- Give a detailed explanation of any proposed pharmacotherapy: Discuss side effects, and agree aims and desired outcomes with the patient.
- Tailor drug to symptom profile of patient: No drug will treat 'the personality disorder' but some drugs may alleviate specific symptoms.
- Specify a few target symptoms and agree how to evaluate them (e.g. a simple rating scale).
- Avoid polypharmacy where possible and evaluate one agent at a time.
- Make a joint plan, specifying agent and duration of trial. Plan review frequency and outline next steps if outcome is unsatisfactory.
- Discontinue medications that have been tried at a satisfactory dose for a reasonable length of time without *any* sign of benefit (6–8 weeks is a good rule of thumb). Gradually reduce the doses of drugs being discontinued.
- Consider potential toxicity and limit prescription size in self-harming patients.

 ## Rapid tranquillisation (RT)

- RT is the use of psychotropic medication to control agitation, threatening or destructive behaviour. Its aim is to calm/lightly sedate the patient in order to reduce risk and allow a thorough psychiatric assessment to take place.
- NICE have published comprehensive guidelines on the short-term management of violence covering a wide range of issues, ranging from environmental and psychosocial aspects such as deescalation, to staff training and post-incident reviews. The updated NICE guideline published in 2015 uses the term RT to refer to parenterally administered medication only.

Environmental and psychological management

- The first steps in dealing with acute behavioural disturbance do not involve drugs.
- The emphasis should be on efforts to 'talk down' the patient while paying common-sense attention to environmental issues and the safety and dignity of the patient, clinical staff and others.
- Even in the most urgent of situations it is important to give due consideration to assessment: Diagnostic, interpersonal and sustaining factors are all relevant.
- Adequate training of all staff is necessary.

Pharmacological management

General considerations

- Although RT is targeted at symptoms/behaviour not the underlying disorder, in many cases in psychiatric services a psychotic disorder will be present, though mania, personality disorder, drug intoxication and general distress can all be important factors.
- Recent emphasis on the desired outcome of RT is the recipient being 'calm and conscious' rather than 'asleep'.
- RT must always be in the context of psychological and environmental management and is not a substitute for it.
- RT is not without risk, whatever the agent used, and safety is a primary consideration. It needs to be balanced against the risk of not adequately treating behavioural disturbance.

- If general, non-pharmacological, measures are ineffective or inappropriate, then oral administration is the first route of choice. Only if this proves impractical should parenteral administration be considered.
- Escalating situations and past history should guide timing of RT; early oral administration may prevent the need for later parenteral drugs.
- A clear treatment plan should be recorded, including timing and dose of subsequent drug administration.
- The management plan should be reviewed regularly and at least every 24 h.
- Wherever possible, the wishes of the patient, including those documented in advance statements, should be determined and respected.

Choice of drugs for rapid tranquillisation

- The choice of agent/s centres on antipsychotics, BDZs or both (see Table 9.3 for drugs commonly used in RT and comments on individual drugs).
- Liquid preparations or disintegrating tablets are useful to ensure absorption when drugs are given orally.
- An antipsychotic is a reasonable choice if it is also an appropriate treatment for an underlying psychotic disorder; otherwise, lorazepam should be considered.
- Combined haloperidol + lorazepam is commonly used clinically in more severe situations in spite of little evidence for benefit over either given individually.
- Overall there is little good quality trial evidence for the efficacy and safety of drugs used in RT. Two Cochrane reviews have compared BDZ with other drugs, and haloperidol with other drugs, for psychosis-induced aggression or agitation:
  - BDZ, antipsychotics and the combination do not significantly differ in efficacy, but BDZ alone causes fewer extrapyramidal side effects (EPSE) and the combination is more sedating.
  - Haloperidol, aripiprazole, olanzapine, risperidone and ziprasidone have similar efficacy but haloperidol causes more EPSE than the rest.
  - Compared with haloperidol, olanzapine is more sedating and ziprasidone causes more cardiac adverse effects.
  - The combination of haloperidol and promethazine (an antihistaminic and antimuscarinic drug) appears more effective than lorazepam or haloperidol alone with fewer EPSE than the latter.
- Parenteral administration
  - Guidelines on parenteral administration abound. A recent review of 45 local UK guidelines in National Health Service organisations found that lorazepam, haloperidol and olanzapine were most commonly recommended drugs for intramuscular use, but other BDZs, antipsychotics, promethazine and paraldehyde were included.

Table 9.3 Drugs in current use for rapid tranquillisation

Drug	Oral	Parenteral	Comments and precautions
Antipsychotics[a]			
Aripiprazole	+	+	Monitor sedation if combined with BDZ.
Chlorprom-azine	+	Do not use	Little RCT evidence. Not recommended by NICE because of cardiac concerns/hypotension.
Haloperidol[b]	+	+	Caution in antipsychotic-naïve patients and with other antipsychotics. ECG advised. Use with anticholinergic. Can be combined with lorazepam if necessary.
Olanzapine	+	+ Use im only	Do not give im within 1 h of intramuscular lorazepam because of concerns about cardiorespiratory depression.
Risperidone	+	NA	
Ziprasidone	+	+	More cardiac effects than haloperidol. Not available in Europe.
Zuclopenthixol acetate (Acuphase)	NA	+ im only	Do not use in antipsychotic naïve patients; only use if repeated im injection/prolonged disturbance/good previous response.
Benzodiazepines			
Diazepam	+	+ Use iv only	Not routinely recommended
Lorazepam[b]	+	+	Dilute with equal volume of sterile saline or water. Do not mix in same syringe as antipsychotic.
Midazolam	Do not use	+	Limited by very short half-life (2–3 h). Can be given buccally. Mixed evidence on efficacy compared with alternatives.
Others			
Promethazine[b]	+	+	Antihistamine. Used safely with haloperidol in large RCTs and may reduce EPSE.
Paraldehyde	Do not use	+ Use im only	Only exceptional use. Avoid more than brief contact with plastic syringe (dissolves plastic).

Consult the British National Formulary and NICE/local guidelines for doses and use in clinical situations.

+, available; BDZ, benzodiazepine; EPSE, extrapyramidal side effects; im, intramuscular; iv, intravenous; NA, not available; RCT, randomised controlled trial.

[a] Antipsychotics are associated with an increased risk of stroke in dementia patients.

[b] Recommended for parenteral use by NICE (2015).

- Particular attention is drawn to cardiac effects and EPSE as important limitations of antipsychotics, particularly if given intravenously (it is debatable whether this is ever warranted). Haloperidol in particular is associated with cardiac effects and the risk of EPSE (if used combined with an anticholinergic drug), so consider the use of a second-generation drug such as olanzapine or aripiprazole.
- The main concern with parenteral BDZs is respiratory depression (especially if other sedative drugs have been taken). Intramuscular lorazepam appears the safest and most practical first-line current option. BDZ-induced disinhibition appears unlikely in the acute situation, but is a possible reason for haloperidol combined with midazolam appearing less effective than other drugs in one RCT.
- Parenteral treatment should only be used if it is possible to undertake careful observation and monitoring, there are resuscitation facilities and flumazenil (BDZ antagonist) is available if lorazepam is used.
- Updated NICE guidance published in 2015 recommends only lorazepam on its own or intramuscular haloperidol together with intramuscular promethazine. Lorazapam should be used if the patient is antipsychotic-naive, has not had an ECG or there evidence of cardiovascular disease.

- It is not uncommon for high doses of drugs to be used either knowingly or inadvertently. When it is necessary to use high doses, consult guidance on high-dose antipsychotic prescribing (e.g. Royal College of Psychiatrists consensus statement – see Guidelines).
- The management of behavioural disturbance extends beyond the acute phase. Planning ongoing pharmacology management is important, as is addressing the impact on the patient and staff.

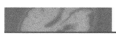

Acknowledgement

This is an update and revision of the third edition chapter which was contributed to by Ian C Reid.

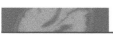

Bibliography

Guidelines

National Institute for Health and Care Excellence. Violence and aggression: Short-term management in mental health, health and community settings. *NICE guideline 10.* 2015; http://www.nice.org.uk/guidance/ng10.

National Institute for Health and Care Excellence. Antisocial personality disorder: Treatment, management and prevention. *NICE Clinical Guideline 77.* 2009; http://www.nice.org.uk/guidance/cg77.

National Institute for Health and Care Excellence. Borderline personality disorder: Treatment and management. *NICE Clinical Guideline 78*. 2009; http://www.nice.org.uk/guidance/cg78.

Royal College of Psychiatrists. Consensus statement on high-dose antipsychotic medication. *Council Report CR190*. 2014; http://www.rcpsych.ac.uk/usefulresources/publications/collegereports/cr/cr190.aspx.

Key references

Bateman AW, Tyrer P. Personality Disorder: No Longer a Diagnosis of Exclusion: PolicyImplementation Guidance for the Development of Services for People with Personality Disorder. Department of Health. 2003; http://www.publications.doh.gov.uk/mentalhealth/personalitydisorder.htm.

Gibbon S, Duggan C, Stoffers JM et al. Psychological interventions for antisocial personality disorder. *Cochrane Database Syst Rev.* 2010(6): CD007668.

Gillies D, Sampson S, Beck A, Rathbone J. Benzodiazepines for psychosis-induced aggression or agitation. *Cochrane Database Syst Rev.* 2013(4): CD003079.

Khalifa N, Duggan C, Lieb K, Stoffers JM, Huband N, Völlm B, Ferriter M. Pharmacological interventions for antisocial personality disorder. *Cochrane Database Syst Rev.* 2010(8): CD007667.

Koenigsberg HW, Reynolds D, Goodman M et al. Risperidone in the treatment of schizotypal personality disorder. *J Clin Psychiatry.* 2003; 64: 628–634.

Powney MJ, Adams CE, Jones H. Haloperidol for psychosis-induced aggression or agitation (rapid tranquillisation). *Cochrane Database Syst Rev.* 2012(11): CD009377.

Stoffers JM, Völlm B, Rücker G, Timmer A, Huband N, Lieb K. Pharmacological interventions for borderline personality disorder. *Cochrane Database Syst Rev.* 2010(6): CD005653.

Stoffers JM, Völlm B, Rücker G, Timmer A, Huband, N, Lieb K. Psychological interventions for borderline personality disorder. *Cochrane Database Syst Rev.* 2012(8): CD005652.

Further reading

Ahmed U, Jones H, Adams CE. Chlorpromazine for psychosis induced aggression or agitation. *Cochrane Database Syst Rev.* 2010(4): CD007445.

American Psychiatric Association. Personality disorders. American Psychiatric Publishing. 2013; http://www.dsm5.org/Documents/Personality%20Disorders%20Fact%20Sheet.pdf.

Baker-Glenn E, Steels M, Evans C. Use of psychotropic medication among psychiatric outpatients with personality disorder. *Psychiatrist.* 2010; 34: 83–86.

Cloninger CR, Svrakic DM, Pryzbeck TR. A psychobiological model of temperament and character. *Arch Gen Psychiatry.* 1993; 50: 975–990.

Innes J, Sehti F. Current rapid tranquillisation documents in the UK: A review of the drugs recommended, the routes of administration and clinical parameters influencing their use. *J Psychiatr Intensive Care.* 2013; 9: 110–118.

Jayakody K, Gibson RC, Kumar A, Gunadasa S. Zuclopenthixol acetate for acute schizophrenia and similar serious mental illnesses. *Cochrane Database Syst Rev.* 2012(4): CD000525.

McAllister-Williams RH, Ferrier IN. Rapid tranquillisation: Time for a reappraisal of options for parenteral therapy. *Br J Psychiatry.* 2002; 180: 485–489.

Taylor D, Paton C, Kapur S. *The Maudsley Prescribing Guidelines in Psychiatry*, 12th edn. Chichester, UK: John Wiley & Sons Ltd., 2015.

Zanarini MC, Frankenburg FR, Hennen J, Silk KR. The longitudinal course of borderline psychopathology: 6-year prospective follow-up of the phenomenology of borderline personality disorder. *Am J Psychiatry* 2003; 160: 274–283.

Drug treatments for child and adolescent disorders

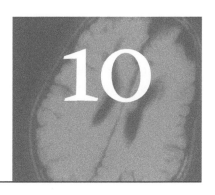

David R Coghill

 ## Background

- Changes in the regulations in both the United States and European Union (EU) have increased clinical trial activity in child and adolescent mental health, but it is still the case that, for many disorders, increased use of medications has tended to outstrip research.
- The consequence is that there is a relative lack of an evidence base on which to make prescribing decisions.
- This is important as children are not simply 'mini-adults'.
  - Their developing brains almost certainly react differently to psychoactive medication.
  - Differences in metabolism make it likely that they will display different side-effect profiles to those seen in adults.

Attention deficit/hyperactivity disorder

- Diagnosis of attention deficit/hyperactivity disorder (ADHD):
  - *DSM-5* requires early onset, pervasive and extreme levels of *inattentive*, *impulsive* and *hyperactive* behaviour, resulting in significant *impairment* and *disability* across settings and unexplained by other disorders.
  - The *ICD-10* diagnosis of *hyperkinetic disorder* is restricted to those with more severe, pervasive and impairing ADHD.
- Epidemiology:
  - Prevalence ~5% (hyperkinetic disorder ~1.5%) and two to three times more likely in boys than girls.
  - Highly comorbid, especially with oppositional defiant disorder and conduct disorder.

- Over diagnosed in many parts of the world (including United States and United Kingdom), but paradoxically still only a small proportion of those with ADHD are correctly identified and treated.
- Course and outcome:
  - A chronic condition that continues through adolescence and into adulthood.
  - When untreated is commonly associated with educational and employment difficulties, relationship problems, increased accidents, substance misuse and delinquency.
  - Recent evidence indicates that treatment reduces symptoms, improves quality of life and decreases functional impairments.

Scientific background

Although the aetiology of ADHD is incompletely understood, increasing evidence strongly supports a biological basis.

Genetic studies

- Heritability of ADHD estimated as greater than 0.7.
- Molecular genetics:
  - Replicated evidence implicating dopamine (DA) genes (D_4, D_5, the DA transporter)
  - Preliminary evidence implicating D_1 and $5-HT_{1B}$, DA-β-hydroxylase and synaptosomal-associated protein 25 (SNAP-25, involved in the regulation of neurotransmitter release)
  - Polygenic with small contribution from each gene (odds ratios [ORs], 1.2–1.9)

Environmental factors

- Evidence for contribution to risk of developing ADHD from
  - Antenatal and perinatal factors (e.g. alcohol, nicotine, low birthweight, obstetric complications, possibly intrauterine valproate exposure)
  - Environmental pollutants such as lead, polychlorinated biphenyls (PCBs) and mercury

Brain imaging and electrophysiology

- Structural/functional abnormalities have been shown in many brain regions including frontal, temporal and parietal cortical regions, basal ganglia, callosal areas and cerebellum.
- Abnormalities are evident early in development, non-progressive and do not appear to be a consequence of stimulant treatment.

Neuropsychology

- Studies demonstrate deficits in higher-order cognitive functions, including working memory and inhibition, motivational processes, as well as more basic aspects of cognition such as spatial memory, timing and time perception.

Neurotransmitters

- Converging evidence for catecholamine dysregulation from
  - Animal models
  - Molecular genetic findings
  - Functional imaging studies
  - The effectiveness of stimulants (DA effects) and NAergic drugs in treatment

Management of ADHD

- Multimodal intervention is usually indicated and should target both the core ADHD symptoms and associated or comorbid problems.
- Psychological and educational interventions, medication and diet should all be available, and their use should be guided by an individualised treatment plan.
- Non-pharmacological treatments include the following:
  - *Psychoeducational measures*: Education and advice should be universal and form the base of any treatment offered.
  - *Parent training and family behavioural interventions*: Many approaches and evidence-based treatment manuals are available. Effectiveness has been shown in individual RCTs but challenged by recent meta-analyses.
  - *Behavioural interventions (preschool or school)*: Effective in reducing hyperactive behaviour and promoting social adjustment with no one scheme shown to be superior to others.

Pharmacological treatments

Stimulant drugs

- These have been used to treat ADHD symptoms since 1937.
- Licensed stimulants in the EU are *methylphenidate, dexamfetamine (dexamphetamine)* and *lisdexamphetamine.*
- Also licensed in the United States *are mixed amphetamine salts* (Adderall®, containing 25% levoamphetamine, 75% dextroamphetamine), *dexmethylphenidate* (the D-isomer of methylphenidate) and *methamphetamine.*

■ Mechanism of action (see also Chapter 1):
  – Methylphenidate is a DA transporter blocker.
  – Dexamphetamine blocks the DA transporter and stimulates synaptic DA release.
  – Lisdexamphetamine is a prodrug for dexamphetamine.
  – Both methylphenidate and dexamphetamine increase DA levels in the nucleus accumbens and therefore have abuse potential (see Chapter 7). However, the best available evidence suggests that treatment of ADHD with stimulants does not increase, and may decrease, the likelihood of later substance misuse.
■ Immediate-release methylphenidate and dexamphetamine have very similar pharmacokinetic, pharmacodynamic and clinical effects:
  – Short half-life ($t_{1/2}$ = 3 h), rapid onset of action (t_{max} = 1.5 h) and short duration of action (3–4 h).
  – Require multiple daily dosing (two or three times per day).
  – Adderall appears to have a longer duration of action than immediate-release methylphenidate from comparative studies.
■ Extended-release methylphenidate preparations increase the duration of action to 8–12 h. The various preparations have different proportions of immediate- and extended-release methylphenidate, offering different bioavailability profiles through the day.
■ Adderall XR is an extended-release preparation based on bead technology and designed to be effective over 12 h.
■ Lisdexamphetamine is inactive until hydrolysed to dexamphetamine. This occurs almost entirely after absorption into red blood cells resulting in a duration of action ~13 h, so that only once-daily administration is required.
■ Efficacy:
  – Short-term efficacy at reducing core ADHD symptoms is established in a large number of RCTs and meta-analyses (large mean effect size ~1.0). Methylphenidate and dexamphetamine are both effective in around 70% of cases; ~95% of patients have a clinically meaningful response to one drug or the other.
  – Adderall may have a small, but statistically significant, efficacy advantage over immediate-release methylphenidate.
  – They are rapidly effective with a response seen after first dose, but require titration to establish most effective dose.
  – Evidence for longer-term efficacy weaker; there are no truly long-term trials of stimulant treatment of ADHD.
■ Adverse effects:
  – *Most common*: Decreased appetite and insomnia, raised blood pressure (all probably dose related)
  – *Less common*: Depression, irritability and increase in tics
  – *Rare*: Rash and allergic reactions, blood dyscrasias and hepatotoxicity, possibly serious cardiovascular events
■ Monitoring of height, weight, pulse and blood pressure recommended
■ Drug interactions (see Table 10.1)

Table 10.1 Selected drug interactions with stimulant drugs

Action/effect	Drug/drug class
Inhibition of metabolism/increased plasma concentration of named drug	TCAs SSRIs Some anticonvulsants (phenobarbital, phenytoin, primidone)
Decreased therapeutic effect of named drugs	Antipsychotics Adrenergic neuron blockers (antihypertensive action)
Hypertension	MAOIs Oxytocin Doxapram
Increased plasma concentration of methylphenidate	Some anticonvulsants (phenobarbital, phenytoin, primidone)
Sudden death (causal link not established)	Clonidine

Atomoxetine

▪ Atomoxetine is licensed in the EU and the United States.
▪ A highly specific NA reuptake inhibitor.
▪ It affects DA as well as NA function and it is likely that clinical effects are associated with both.
▪ No alteration of DA levels in the nucleus accumbens; thus is unlikely to be associated with abuse potential.
▪ Metabolised by hepatic CYP2D6, but no association between poor metaboliser status and increased adverse events reported.
▪ Efficacy:
  – Published RCTs (all industry-sponsored) reported atomoxetine superior to placebo in reduction of core ADHD symptoms in all ages (mean effect size 0.7).
  – RCTs comparing atomoxetine and stimulants are difficult to interpret due to the design of the studies; however, stimulants appear to have the greater effect size.
  – Although plasma $t_{1/2}$ of atomoxetine is short (~4 h), the behavioural effects last longer than predicted from this, with sustained effects through the day with once-daily dosing.
  – Effects may be seen early but continue to increase over several weeks; for some patients, maximum effects appear to take several months.
▪ Adverse effects:
  – Most common are decreased appetite, vomiting, nausea, dizziness, asthenia and dyspepsia.

- – Possible increased risk of seizures.
- – An increased risk of suicidal thinking has been found in short-term studies in children with ADHD, but not in adults.
- ▦ Indications:
  - – Usually after non-response to, or failure to tolerate, stimulant treatment.
  - – May be considered first line where coexisting substance misuse, a need to control symptoms in the late evening or early morning or a desire to avoid stimulants.

Guanfacine and clonidine

- ▦ Extended-release preparations of guanfacine and clonidine are licensed in the United States, with studies ongoing with a guanfacine preparation in Europe.
- ▦ Both are α_2-adrenoceptor agonists, originally developed as antihypertensives.
- ▦ Efficacy: A meta-analysis of 11 clonidine trials found a moderate effect size of 0.58.
- ▦ Adverse effects:
  - – Most common: Sleepiness, tiredness, trouble sleeping, low blood pressure, nausea, stomach pain and dizziness.
  - – Less common: Fainting due to low heart rate and hypotension low heart rate and fainting.
- ▦ While both are efficacious as stand-alone treatments, their clinical place is probably as adjuncts to stimulant preparations.

Modafinil

- ▦ Licensed to improving wakefulness in patients with excessive sleepiness associated with narcolepsy, obstructive sleep apnoea and shift work sleep disorder.
  - – Plans to license it for ADHD were halted after reports of rare but serious skin reactions (including suspected erythema multiforme and Steven–Johnson syndrome).
  - – Promotes wakefulness that is distinct from amphetamines; considered by some to be a cognitive enhancer.
- ▦ Mechanism of action is unclear and includes possible DA transporter inhibition, activation of orexin-containing neurons, histamine release and altering glutamate: GABA neuronal balance. Also proposed are
  - – Action on brain sites involved in 'normal' wakefulness, including hypothalamus, without generalised CNS excitation.
  - – Enhancement of hypothalamo–cortical pathways resulting in maintenance of prefrontal cortical activity involved in higher-order executive functions, motor-sensory coordination and goal-directed behaviours.

- Demonstrated efficacy in treating ADHD in three industry-sponsored RCTs (mean effect size 0.7).
- *Main side effects*: Insomnia, headache, appetite decrease and abdominal pain.
- Low abuse potential.

Tricyclic antidepressants (see Chapter 4)

- Previously recommended in the United Kingdom as third-line treatment for ADHD, now less frequently used since the introduction of atomoxetine.
- Tricyclic antidepressants (TCAs) are associated with a wide range of side effects, are toxic in overdose and should be used with extreme caution in children and adolescents.
- In terms of efficacy, a systematic review concluded that
  - Studies comparing stimulants with TCAs have many limitations.
  - Desipramine is more effective than placebo (withdrawn from the market in the United Kingdom due to concerns over cardiotoxicity).
  - Evidence for imipramine is insufficient with inconsistent results.

Prescribing issues and clinical guidance for treating ADHD

- Despite continuing public and media controversy there is little evidence that stimulants or atomoxetine lead to negative long-term outcomes (studies are ongoing to establish this with more certainty).
- Large inter individual variation with stimulants requires careful dose titration to balance symptom reduction and side effects.
- Longer-acting stimulant preparations, avoiding the need to take medication three times a day (including at school), appear to reduce non-adherence, stigma and restriction in activities.
- The need for medication in ADHD is an individual decision, but non-pharmacological measures alone are unlikely to be sufficient for more severe cases (e.g. *ICD-10* hyperkinetic disorder).
- The UK NICE guideline recommends methylphenidate as a first-line drug treatment for ADHD (Scottish Intercollegiate Guidelines Network also recommend dexamphetamine) and lisdexamphetamine and atomoxetine for those who do not achieve an optimal response. Prescribing is subject to specialist initiation and management and shared care with primary care.
- The influential Multimodal Treatment Study of ADHD (MTA study) demonstrated the superiority of a carefully managed and structured medication package over both behavioural treatment and unstructured community-based pharmacological treatment. Components included

more intensive medication regime, blind initial dose titration, supportive counselling and reading materials and monthly consultations for dose adjustment.

Autism spectrum disorder

- In *DSM-5*, the various aspects of autism are brought together in the single diagnosis of autism spectrum disorder (ASD), the core features of which are deficits in social and communicative functioning with repetitive behaviours, interests and activities.
- Its complex aetiology is poorly understood but there is evidence for reduced 5-HT, and altered DA, neurotransmission.
- Educational and behavioural treatments remain the mainstay of treatment for children and adolescents with ASD.

Drug treatments for ASD

- There are no effective pharmacological treatments for the core symptoms of ASD.
- Medication may play an adjunctive role for specific behaviours such as hyperactivity, aggression, withdrawal and repetitive, ritualised, stereotyped or self-injurious behaviours.

Antipsychotics (see Chapter 3)

Critics suggest that antipsychotics are used merely as 'chemical straitjackets', but particularly for the atypical antipsychotics, this is not borne out by the evidence.

Typical antipsychotics

- Haloperidol has been the most studied drug in autism.
- Evidence from RCTs shows efficacy in reducing a wide range of maladaptive behaviours (including hyperactivity, withdrawal, aggression and temper tantrums, stereotypes, mood lability), increasing social relatedness and discriminant learning.
- However, adverse effects are frequent and disabling:
  - Short-term: Excessive sedation and extrapyramidal side effects (EPSE) are common.
  - Withdrawal dyskinesias are suffered by about 1/3, and tardive dyskinesia by ~10%, of children.
- Despite proven effectiveness, the adverse effects severely limit the use of haloperidol in autism.

Atypical antipsychotics

- Risperidone and aripiprazole are licensed in the United States for the treatment of irritability and aggression in ASD.
- Efficacy (independent of common adverse events such as drowsiness and fatigue) has been demonstrated for
  - Aggression and irritability: Effect size ~1.2 for risperidone and 0.6–0.9 for aripiprazole used in low dose (RCT data also support the efficacy of olanzapine and quetiapine)
  - Tantrums, aggression and self-injurious behaviour
  - Reduction of stereotypies and repetitive behaviours
- Adverse effects:
  - Relatively common: Increased appetite and weight gain, fatigue, drowsiness, dizziness and drooling.
  - EPSE are not common, but more frequent than in adults.

Other medications

- *Methylphenidate, atomoxetine*: Supported by clinical guidelines to treat ADHD symptoms (ADHD is frequently comorbid).
- *Selective serotonin reuptake inhibitors (SSRIs)*: May benefit anxiety symptoms based on clinical experience, but good trial data are lacking.
- *Fluvoxamine*: Conflicting data. One RCT found efficacy in reducing repetitive thoughts and behaviour, maladaptive behaviour and aggression and improving some aspects of social relatedness, particularly language use. Another RCT reported no benefit over placebo.
- *Fluoxetine, clomipramine, valproate*: Statistically significant, but not clinically important, reduction in stereotypies and repetitive behaviours has been reported.

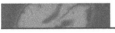 **Depressive disorders** (see Chapter 4)

Antidepressants

Antidepressants have been the subject of extreme scrutiny, with concerns raised questioning both their safety and efficacy:

Tricyclic antidepressants

- TCAs do not appear to be effective and should not be used in the treatment of depression in prepubertal children.
- There is marginal evidence to support the use of TCAs in the treatment of depression in adolescents, but benefits are likely to be moderate at best.
- Side effects and toxicity in overdose mean extreme caution is required in their use.

SSRIs and other serotonergic drugs

- Fluoxetine is licensed for depression in children over the age of 8 in the United States and EU, with escitalopram also licensed for children over 12 in the United States.
- Efficacy is less well established in children and adolescents than in adults:
  - *Fluoxetine*: Consistently positive RCTs
  - *Sertraline, citalopram, escitalopram*: Mixed results
  - *Paroxetine, venlafaxine, nefazodone, mirtazapine*: Negative results
- The effect size is smaller than in adults, with larger placebo effects. One meta-analysis of RCTs of SSRI found a pooled response OR against placebo of 1.57 for the SSRIs (OR 2.39 for fluoxetine, the only drug individually to show benefit), and another reported the number needed to treat (NNT) as 14 for children under 12 and 8 for adolescents.
- Nevertheless, two large, publically funded, studies investigating the comparative effectiveness of SSRI and CBT found SSRIs effective. The efficacy of CBT was less obvious, and it is still unclear whether adding CBT to SSRI improves outcome.
- Both the UK and US regulatory authorities warn about an increased risk of suicidal thoughts and behaviour in patients under 18 years of age (~4% vs. ~2% on placebo); however, an increased risk of completed suicide has not been demonstrated.

Clinical guidance

- Psychotherapy, particularly cognitive behavioural therapy (CBT) and interpersonal therapy (IPT), is effective and generally recommended as first-line treatment for depression in children and adolescents.
- Antidepressants are indicated for moderate to severe depressive disorders in adolescents where effective psychosocial interventions are impractical or where depression fails to respond to an adequate trial of psychotherapy of at least 3 months.
- The clinical benefit of antidepressants is less certain for children under 12 years.
- They should not be used as the sole intervention and only initiated after specialist consultation.
- In practice ~60% of young people with depression will respond adequately to initial treatment with an SSRI. Switching to another SSRI and/or adding CBT is beneficial for many of those not responding to the first SSRI.

- NICE (2015) guidance on treating depression in children and young people recommends:
  - Considering combined fluoxetine and psychological therapy as an initial treatment of moderate to severe depression in young people (12–18 years) as an alternative to psychological therapy alone.
  - Fluoxetine for first line antidepressant in cases of moderate or severe depression unresponsive to psychological intervention after 4–6 sessions.
  - Cautiously considering the use of fluoxetine to treat moderate to severe depression in younger children (5–11 years) who have not responded to a specific psychological therapy after 4 to 6 sessions.
  - If fluoxetine is not effective or tolerated, then sertraline and citalopram are recommended as second-line.
  - Consideration of atypical antipsychotic augmentation in psychotic depression.
  - Antidepressants should be continued for at least 6 months after remission.
  - Paroxetine, venlafaxine and TCAs should not be prescribed.

Manic episodes and bipolar disorder (see Chapter 5)

- There is uncertainty and disagreement about the diagnosis of manic episodes and bipolar disorder (BD) in child and adolescent populations. In the United Kingdom, a diagnosis of BD is still rarely made, but it is much more common in the United States, often as bipolar-II disorder or bipolar disorder not otherwise specified (NOS).
- The nature of patients included in clinical trials, and whether clinicians would recognise them as having BD, is uncertain, which makes the evidence base difficult to interpret and translation into clinical practice problematic.
- Nevertheless 'true' manic episodes in children and adolescents are difficult to treat without medication.
- In the EU, aripiprazole is the only licensed drug for the acute treatment of mania in adolescents with bipolar I disorder. In the United States, aripiprazole, risperidone, quetiapine and olanzapine are licensed for mania in adolescents and lithium for its treatment and prevention.
- A systematic review and meta-analysis of drug treatment of mania in children and adolescents found a significant overall OR of 2.23:
  - This was mainly accounted for by atypical antipsychotics, with positive RCT evidence for aripiprazole, olanzapine, quetiapine, risperidone and ziprasidone.
  - Topiramate and oxcarbazepine had lesser effect, and valproate was ineffective.

▓ NICE (2014) bipolar clinical guidelines recommend aripiprazole for mania in adolescents and to also consider the recommendations for adults (see Chapter 5). Valproate should be avoided in girls of child-bearing potential (see Chapter 11).

Obsessive–compulsive disorder (see Chapter 6)

▓ While CBT and exposure with response prevention remain first-line treatments for early-onset obsessive–compulsive disorder (OCD), there is a good evidence base to support the use of medication.
▓ The SSRIs have been demonstrated to be safe and effective treatments for paediatric OCD. Sertraline and fluvoxamine are licensed for use in children and adolescents in the EU and the United States. Fluoxetine and clomipramine are also licensed in the United States.
▓ Clomipramine is effective but safety issues limit its usefulness in clinical practice.
▓ Long-term treatment is well tolerated and effective at maintaining improvement, with continued improvement seen for up to 1 year.
▓ Obsessional symptoms may relapse on discontinuation of treatment; it is suggested that treatment withdrawal should be attempted 1–1.5 years after symptom resolution and restarted if significant symptoms reoccur.
▓ Paediatric OCD may not respond as well to some SSRIs as does adult OCD: A course of treatment results in 20%–25% being symptom-free, 20%–50% with some improvement and ~25% with no improvement.

Anxiety disorders (see Chapter 6)

▓ The use of drug treatments in the management of anxiety in children and adolescents is contentious; many clinicians argue that only psychosocial interventions should be used.
▓ However, success rates for CBT are 70%–80%, so a significant proportion of children will require further intervention.

Antidepressants

▓ None are licensed in this age group for this indication.
▓ The SSRIs are now the first-choice pharmacological treatment for child and adolescent anxiety disorders.

- Fluvoxamine, fluoxetine, sertraline, paroxetine and venlafaxine have all been reported to be efficacious in short-term RCTs in treating paediatric generalised anxiety disorder with a pooled NNT of four in children and two in adolescents and effect sizes ranging from 0.5 to 1.5.
- RCTs of TCAs conducted in paediatric anxiety have not demonstrated clear efficacy. This, together with their adverse effects, means they are not indicated for these disorders.

Benzodiazepines

- Generally efficacious, however, adverse events and risk of tolerance mean that they should only be considered when other pharmacological approaches have failed and should only be prescribed for very short periods of time.

Buspirone

- Several open-label studies suggest buspirone is comparable in efficacy to the benzodiazepines in childhood anxiety disorders, with fewer adverse events. However, controlled data are lacking.

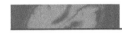 **Bibliography**

Guidelines

Bolea-Alamanac B, Nutt DJ, Adamou M. et al. Evidence-based guidelines for the pharmacological management of attention deficit hyperactivity disorder: Update on recommendations from the British Association for Psychopharmacology. *J Psychopharmacol.* 2014; 28: 179–203. http://bap.org.uk/pdfs/ADHD_Guidelines.pdf.

National Institute for Health and Care Excellence. Depression in children and young people: Identification and management in primary, community and secondary care. *NICE Clinical Guideline 28.* 2015; https://www.nice.org.uk/guidance/cg28.

National Institute for Health and Care Excellence. Attention deficit hyperactivity disorder: Diagnosis and management of ADHD in children, young people and adults. *NICE clinical guideline 72.* 2008; https://www.nice.org.uk/guidance/cg72.

National Institute for Health and Care Excellence. Aripiprazole for treating moderate to severe manic episodes in adolescents with bipolar I disorder. *NICE Technology Appraisal Guidance 292.* 2013; http://www.nice.org.uk/guidance/TA292.

National Institute for Health and Care Excellence. Autism: The management and support of children and young people on the autism spectrum. *NICE Clinical Guideline 170.* 2013; https://www.nice.org.uk/guidance/cg170.

National Institute for Health and Care Excellence. Bipolar disorder: The assessment and management of bipolar disorder in adults, children and young people in primary and secondary care. *NICE Clinical Guideline 185.* 2014; https://www.nice.org.uk/guidance/cg185.

Key references

Banaschewski T, Coghill D, Santosh P et al. Long-acting medications for the hyperkinetic disorders: A systematic review and European treatment guideline. *Eur Child Adolesc Psychiatry.* 2006; 15: 476–495.

Brent D, Emslie G, Clarke G et al. Switching to another SSRI or to venlafaxine with or without cognitive behavioral therapy for adolescents with SSRI-resistant depression: The TORDIA randomized controlled trial. *JAMA.* 2008; 299: 901–913.

Bridge JA, Iyengar S, Salary CB et al. Clinical response and risk for reported suicidal ideation and suicide attempts in pediatric antidepressant treatment: A meta-analysis of randomized controlled trials. *JAMA.* 2007; 297: 1683–1696.

Cortese S, Holtmann M, Banaschewski T et al. Current best practice in the management of adverse events during treatment with ADHD medications in children and adolescents. *J Child Psychol Psychiatry.* 2013; 54: 227–246.

Emslie GJ, Mayes T, Porta G et al. Treatment of resistant depression in adolescents (TORDIA): Week 24 outcomes. *Am J Psychiatry.* 2010; 167: 782–791.

Faraone SV, Buitelaar J. Comparing the efficacy of stimulants for ADHD in children and adolescents using meta-analysis. *Eur Child Adolesc Psychiatry.* 2010; 19: 353–364.

Goodyer I, Dubicka B, Wilkinson P et al. Selective serotonin reuptake inhibitors (SSRIs) and routine specialist care with and without cognitive behaviour therapy in adolescents with major depression: Randomised controlled trial. *BMJ.* 2007; 335: 142.

Jensen PS, Arnold LE, Swanson JM et al. 3-year follow-up of the NIMH MTA study. *J Am Acad Child Adolesc Psychiatry.* 2007; 46: 989–1002.

Liu HY, Potter MP, Woodworth KY et al. Pharmacologic treatments for pediatric bipolar disorder: A review and meta-analysis. *J Am Acad Child Adolesc Psychiatry.* 2011; 50: 749–762.

March J, Silva S, Petrycki S et al. Fluoxetine, cognitive-behavioral therapy, and their combination for adolescents with depression: Treatment for Adolescents with Depression Study (TADS) randomized controlled trial. *JAMA.* 2004; 292: 807–820.

McDougle CJ, Scahill L, Aman MG et al. Risperidone for the core symptom domains of autism: Results from the study by the autism network of the research units on pediatric psychopharmacology. *Am J Psychiatry.* 2005; 162: 1142–1148.

Usala T, Clavenna A, Zuddas A et al. Randomised controlled trials of selective serotonin reuptake inhibitors in treating depression in children and adolescents: A systematic review and meta-analysis. *Eur Neuropsychopharm.* 2008; 18: 62–73.

Watson HJ, Rees CS. Meta-analysis of randomized, controlled treatment trials for pediatric obsessive–compulsive disorder. *J Child Psychol Psychiatry.* 2008; 49: 489–498.

Further reading

Coghill D, Bonnar S, Duke S et al. *Child and Adolescent Psychiatry (Oxford Specialist Handbooks in Psychiatry).* Oxford, UK: Oxford University Press, 2009.

Coghill D, Sinita E. Pharmacology for ADHD, Tourette syndrome and autism spectrum disorder. In Huline-Dickens S (Ed.). *Clinical Topics in Child and Adolescent Psychiatry.* London, UK: RCPsych Publications, 2014; pp. 74–93.

Hazell P, Mirzaie M. Tricyclic drugs for depression in children and adolescents. *Cochrane Database Syst Rev.* 2013; 6: CD002317.

McVoy M, Findling R (Eds.). *Clinical Manual of Child and Adolescent Psychopharmacology.* Arlington, TX: American Psychiatric Publishing, 2012.

Royal Pharmaceutical Society of Great Britain and British Medical Association. *British National Formulary for Children: 2014–2015*. London, UK: BMJ Group, Pharmaceutical Press, RCPCH, 2014.

Sinita E, Coghill D. Pharmacology for anxiety and obsessive compulsive disorders, affective disorders and schizophrenia. In Huline-Dickens S (Ed.). *Clinical Topics in Child and Adolescent Psychiatry*. London, UK: RCPsych Publications, 2014; pp. 94–111.

Swanson J, Arnold LE, Kraemer H et al. Evidence, interpretation, and qualification from multiple reports of long-term outcomes in the Multimodal Treatment Study of Children with ADHD (MTA). Part I: Executive summary. *J Atten Disord*. 2008; 12: 4–14.

Swanson J, Arnold LE, Kraemer H et al. Evidence, interpretation, and qualification from multiple reports of long-term outcomes in the Multimodal Treatment Study of Children with ADHD (MTA). Part II: Supporting details. *J Atten Disord*. 2008; 12: 15–43.

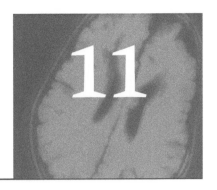

Prescribing in clinical practice

Peter M Haddad and Angelika Wieck

 **Introduction**

- The increased prevalence of depressive and anxiety disorders in patients with chronic medical conditions, and the increased risk of physical illness (e.g. diabetes and cardiovascular disease) in those with psychiatric disorders, means that practitioners in all branches of medicine need to be able to prescribe and monitor psychotropic drugs.
- In addition, there is an increasing tendency for psychiatric conditions to be managed in general medical setting, including by non-medical prescribers, so that knowledge about the basic principles of prescribing, and management of adverse effects, is widely applicable.
- The principles of prescribing outlined in this chapter will apply to most situations, but especially those where particular care is needed, such as the management of the elderly and physically ill. In addition, given its importance, and particular difficulties, we specifically discuss prescribing in pregnancy and lactation.
- Detailing the range of adverse effects is beyond the remit of this chapter; however, more detailed information is given in the relevant chapters in this book, as well as available from review articles and textbooks.

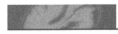 **Phases of treatment**

- The drug treatment of most psychiatric disorders can be broadly divided into acute and longer-term treatment; however, in practice the distinction may not be straightforward.
- *Acute treatment*
  - The goal is full resolution of the illness (complete symptomatic relief and functional recovery), but incomplete remission is not uncommon.
  - There is no fixed length of acute treatment which often merges into longer-term treatment.

- The management of incomplete remission will differ depending on the history of the illness and treatment goals, ranging from treatment sequencing to persisting with current treatment and working with the improvement gained.
- In fluctuating conditions, or with recurrent relapse in chronic conditions, taking a strict acute treatment approach may not be helpful, and the impact on overall illness course may be a better guide.

- *Longer-term treatment* includes:
  - *Continuation treatment*, which is the time-limited use of medication after acute treatment to prevent relapse, with the length of time varying between conditions, but typically at least 6–12 months.
  - *Maintenance treatment*, which is usually for longer periods or indefinitely. This ranges from treatment to prevent relapse (prophylaxis) in recurrent disorders with full remission in between episodes to improving the illness course by minimising residual symptom severity and the severity and frequency of full illness episodes.
  - Drug dosing during longer-term treatment should be at the effective treatment dose if at all possible, and the older concept of a lower 'maintenance dose' lacks an evidence base and is risky.

- It is important to explain and jointly decide with the patient about the phase of treatment and its management, because
  - Treatment that is tolerated in the short-term may not be acceptable longer term (e.g. sexual side effects or weight gain).
  - It can be difficult for patients to adjust to the implications of longer-term treatment, especially if remission is complete, as this requires acceptance of the need for ongoing illness management and of the risk of relapse.

- Stopping treatment always needs planning in consultation with the patient after assessment of relapse/recurrence risk (see Principle 10 in the following text for its management).

Ten principles of good psychiatric prescribing

Principle 1: Ensure the benefits outweigh the risks

- The benefits of a patient taking a drug should outweigh the risks of
  - *No treatment* or *watchful waiting*. For example, in patients with mild depressive symptoms of recent onset, the spontaneous improvement rate is high.
  - *Adverse effects* and *safety*, not only short term, but longer term (e.g. weight gain on mirtazapine, sexual side effects on SSRIs). Treatment should only be started mindful that treatment comprises an acute and a continuation phase (see earlier); therefore,

minimum planned treatment duration for anxiety, depressive and psychotic episodes varies between 9 and 18 months.

- *Alternative treatments*. These include not only alternative drugs but also psychological treatments which may range from low-intensity psychosocial interventions to high-intensity psychotherapy. For many non-psychotic disorders, psychological treatments are as effective as drugs and may be the option of first choice (e.g. some anxiety disorders, or if a medical condition makes drugs more risky). In addition, they often have the advantage of persistent benefit in preventing relapse (e.g. CBT for depression). However, psychological interventions are more difficult to access, take up and completion may be low, costs may be higher, and their quality can be difficult to guarantee.

▨ Determining the risk–benefit balance of pharmacological treatment requires a good knowledge of the evidence base for different treatments including correct dosage and interactions. It needs accurate assessment of the patient including medical history, currently prescribed and over-the-counter medications (including herbal remedies) and good clinical judgement.

▨ Ineffective medication should be discontinued.

▨ Some factors to consider in prescribing safely are summarised in Table 11.1.

Principle 2: Involve the patient in treatment decisions

▨ Where possible, decisions about medication should be jointly made by the clinician and patient in collaboration. This includes patients with impaired capacity or detained under mental health legislation.

▨ The clinician needs to
- Provide the patient with information about their illness
- Discuss the different treatment options, including benefits and potential adverse effects
- Listen to the patient and ascertain and address their treatment aims, concerns and misconceptions

▨ While encouraging participation in shared decision-making is essential, this does not mean simply doing what the patient wants (e.g. if it might be harmful or not effective), nor abrogating professional responsibility for the decision.

Principle 3: Where possible prescribe within licence

▨ Medication can broadly be prescribed as
- *Licensed* when it is used within its marketing authorisation in the country concerned

Table 11.1 Factors to consider in making safe prescribing decisions

Patient age
  Elderly and children/adolescents are more vulnerable to many side effects.
  In these groups, use lower doses and slower titrations.

Is the patient pregnant or likely to become pregnant? If yes
  Obtain expert advice.
  Consider the mother's previous pharmacological treatment history.
  Avoid known teratogens (e.g. lithium, valproate, carbamazepine).
  Choose a drug where there is evidence of safety in pregnancy.
  Consider adverse effects on foetus and newborn other than teratogenesis
    (e.g. impairment of IQ with valproate).
  Consider risk to newborn if subsequent plans to breastfeed while maternal
    prescribing continues.
  Consider risks to mother and unborn child if psychiatric illness is not treated
    pharmacologically.

Are there coexisting medical disorders? In particular consider[a]
  Cardiovascular disease
  Epilepsy
  Renal impairment
  Hepatic impairment
  Respiratory disease
  Gastrointestinal disorders
  Dementia and cerebrovascular disease

Is there a potential for drug interactions?[a,b]
  With other prescribed medication
  With over-the-counter medication
  With alcohol
  With illicit drugs

Is the patient at risk of overdose?
  Consider prescribing a less toxic drug.
  Consider dispensing in limited quantities.
  Consider asking a relative to give our medication (if the patient agrees).

Is there a history of drug allergies or serious drug side effects?
  If so, avoid these or similar drugs.

Source: Adapted from Haddad PM. *Medicine* 2012; 40: 674.

[a] Comorbidity and pharmacodynamic interactions with coprescribed drugs may increase susceptibility to adverse effects and require dose reduction or avoidance of certain drugs.

[b] Pharmacokinetic interactions with coprescribed medication may necessitate either dose reduction or dose decrease.

- – *Unlicensed* when a drug is not marketed for any indication in the country concerned
- – *Off-label* when a licensed drug is used in a different way to that stated its marketing authorisation (this is under the general category of unlicensed use by the General Medical Council, United Kingdom)
- Medications prescribed within their licence have been assessed during licensing as having a favourable balance between benefits and risks for the stated indications, doses and patient population.
- Off-label prescribing is fairly frequent in specialist care where complexity, treatment resistance and special populations are common.
- Unlicensed prescribing, which requires special import into the country, is less so, but may be appropriate (e.g. for a foreign visitor taking a drug licensed in their own country).
- The four main types of off-label prescribing are a drug being used outside of its
  - – Indication
  - – Age group or gender
  - – Dose
  - – Duration
- Off-label prescribing can be appropriate or inappropriate:
  - – Rigidly sticking to licence may limit patient choice, reduce the chance of optimal clinical outcomes and deny a patient a treatment which is supported by a reasonable evidence base.
  - – But poorly thoughtout, off-label prescribing can be ineffective and dangerous.
- Medical practitioners are permitted to prescribe unlicensed and off-label drugs if it is necessary to meet the medical needs of a patient. However,
  - – It should only be conducted within their area of expertise.
  - – There should be an evidence base to support its use.
  - – They take a greater personal responsibility, including overseeing care and ensuring monitoring and follow-up.
  - – As a rule patients should give informed consent, and this should be documented in the notes, together with the reasons for prescribing off-label. A grey area is prescribing alternative and safe drugs within the same class for a disorder where they do not have a licence, but others in class do (e.g. SSRIs in anxiety disorders).
- Drug licenses can differ between countries, a drug may have different approved dose ranges in different indications, and licences can change over time. Consult local prescribing guidance about this, for example, the British National Formulary in the United Kingdom.

Principle 4: Ensure that medication is part of an overall treatment plan

- Always combine medication with monitoring and psychosocial strategies.
- These include the following:
  - Monitoring progress with standardised scales where possible (e.g. Beck Depression Inventory [BDI], Patient Health Questionnaire-9 [PHQ-9]), or target symptoms
  - Education and advice about daily activities, identifying and avoiding or resolving stressors, tackling maladaptive behaviours such as alcohol or substance use, healthy diet, exercise
  - Low- or high-intensity psychological treatments
  - Community nurse, support worker or social worker input

Principle 5: Start with a low dose and increase gradually

- It is not possible to predict at what dose an individual patient will respond, and many modern drugs do not have a clear dose–response efficacy within their licensed doses (e.g. SSRIs).
- Conversely side effects are usually dose related.
- Adaptation to many side effects occurs over days to weeks, so gradual dose increase often reduces their frequency and severity.
- Consider timing doses to minimise impact of adverse effects (e.g. give more sedative drugs at night, alerting ones in the morning).
- Starting with very low doses should be considered in populations particularly prone to drug adverse effects including
  - The elderly or children
  - Medical conditions especially hepatic or renal impairment
  - Previous or likely poor tolerance (e.g. panic disorder with SSRIs)
  - Potential interactions with other drugs, or disorders (e.g. epilepsy)
- However, it is important that this principle does not inadvertently leave a patient on a subtherapeutic dose of medication.

Principle 6: Ensure a therapeutic trial of sufficient duration

- It often takes several weeks between starting an accepted therapeutic dose of a drug and observing a clinically obvious response.
- Response may develop over time so it is important to assess the trajectory of improvement when considering altering treatment.
- Regular follow-up and monitoring. Standardised symptom assessments are recommended for depression in NICE guidelines and are

associated with better treatment response, although few clinicians use them.
- Longer trials of treatment may be indicated in the elderly, and if there has been previous failed response.

Principle 7: Manage adverse effects appropriately

- Adverse effects may cause suffering, impair quality of life, stigmatise patients, lead to non-adherence and, in some cases, be medically serious.
- The management of adverse effects involves
  - The discussion of common, and rare but serious, side effects, with the patient prior to commencing medication
  - Systematic screening for adverse effects during treatment
  - Offering appropriate management when adverse effects are recognised
- Patients who are warned of potential side effects appear less likely to unilaterally stop a medication if they occur.
- Adverse effects should be systematically elicited rather than waiting for the patient to volunteer information. These can be administered, or preferably patient completed (e.g. while waiting for appointments). An example is the Systematic Monitoring of Adverse events Related to Treatments (SMARTS) to assess antipsychotic side effects (Table 11.2).
- Medication-specific monitoring, including blood tests (e.g. lithium) and physical health assessments (e.g. antipsychotics), is often indicated (see relevant chapters).
- Management of adverse effects requires discussion with the patient, weighing them against benefits from the medication and taking appropriate action which includes
  - Reassurance and time, especially for mild transient effects (e.g. early nausea with SSRIs)
  - Lifestyle or symptomatic advice (e.g. dietary advice for weight gain).
  - Change in drug timing or dosage
  - Stopping or switching medication
  - Less often, adding a drug to counteract the effect (e.g. sildenafil for sexual dysfunction, anticholinergics for extrapyramidal side effects)
  - Rarely, urgent intervention for medically serious adverse events (e.g. lithium toxicity, severe allergic reactions)

Principle 8: Avoid unnecessary polypharmacy

- Polypharmacy here refers to combining drugs for treatment of the same disorder (Note: Taking multiple drug treatments for different pathologies carries similar risks).

Table 11.2 Systematic Monitoring of Adverse events Related to Treatments (SMARTS) questionnaire

Instructions

We want to be sure that you are receiving the best treatment and would like to check whether you have any problems which may result from taking your medications.

Please circle any of the following items that trouble you, so that your doctor or nurse can discuss them with you.

Are you troubled by

1. Difficulties in your movement such as shaking, stiffness or muscle aches?
2. Changes in your weight or appetite?
3. Problems with your sex life?
4. Changes in your periods or changes in your breasts?
5. Dizziness or light-headedness?
6. Tiredness or sleepiness?
7. Restlessness or feeling fidgety?
8. Constipation, diarrhoea, nausea, stomach problems or dry mouth?
9. Difficulty passing water or passing water very frequently?
10. Problems with your concentration or memory?
11. Feeling anxious or depressed?
12. Any other problems which you think may be related to your medication?

Please state_____

Source: Haddad PM et al., *Ther Adv Psychopharmacol* 2014a; 4: 15.

- Adverse events are more likely when multiple drugs are used, and interactions can be unpredictable.
- Combining drugs from the same pharmacological class is rarely indicated, except when cross-tapering when switching drugs.
- Combining drugs can be rational when their pharmacological actions are complementary, although the side effect burden is usually higher. Examples include
  - Quetiapine augmentation of SSRIs to treat depression where there is good RCT evidence
  - A second antipsychotic with clozapine for poor response in treatment-resistant schizophrenia
- If a second drug is added to counteract an adverse effect
  - Strong justification is needed for not swapping drug if drugs are from the same broad class (e.g. aripiprazole to reduce raised prolactin caused by another antipsychotic)

- A careful weighing of risks and benefits if they are from different classes (e.g. antimuscarinic drugs for EPSE on antipsychotics)
- Polypharmacy requires pharmacological expertise and should usually be supervised by a specialist.

Principle 9: Explore adherence regularly

- Reviews suggest that over half of patients adhere poorly, or not at all, to medication.
- Non-adherence is often covert and can lead to poorer outcome, e.g. relapse and rehospitalisation in schizophrenia.
- Adherence is likely to be improved by many of the principles of good prescribing already discussed earlier.
- It is important to explore medication adherence regularly and in a non-judgemental way, in order to help guide treatment and avoid inappropriate prescribing decisions being taken.
- Explore non-adherence as a cause of poor response to treatment.

Principle 10: Withdraw medication gradually

- When psychiatric drugs are withdrawn after being taken for at least a few weeks, tapering the drug down over several weeks decreases the likelihood of discontinuation symptoms occurring.
- Symptoms related to discontinuation can be understood in terms of physiological/pharmacological adaptation and rebound following drug withdrawal, and they are recognised with many drugs, not only with psychotropics.
- Discontinuation symptoms are distinguished from addiction-related withdrawal symptoms by the lack of other features of the addiction syndrome (craving, previous dose escalation or tolerance, behaviours to maintain supplies, etc.). Addiction is found with some drugs such as benzodiazepines (see Chapter 6), but rarely if ever with antidepressants and antipsychotics. However, this distinction is seen as a fine one by many people. See Chapter 4 for the discussion of antidepressant discontinuation symptoms.
- Situations where abrupt discontinuation of medication is indicated, or reasonable, include the following:
  - Severe, or medically serious adverse effects (e.g. lithium toxicity), but monitor carefully for 'rebound' illness.
  - Switching from one drug to another in the same class or with similar pharmacological effects.
  - Only brief exposure to the drug (less than a few weeks).
- After complete discontinuation of all drugs, consider risk of relapse, and need for monitoring, and advise the patient about these.

Prescribing in pregnancy and lactation

- Mental ill health is common in pregnancy with at least 1 in 10 women affected. Although non-pharmacological treatments are appropriate for many, women with more severe or complex illnesses often require continued psychotropic medication.
- Childbirth is a powerful trigger for recurrences or new onsets of severe illnesses (particularly manic and psychotic episodes); they often present as psychiatric emergencies and require urgent treatment.
- There is increasing evidence that untreated maternal mental illness can have adverse effects on obstetric and infant outcomes.
- Particular difficulties in prescribing for this patient group include concerns about effects on the foetus, the lack of evidence, and because no drugs are licensed. Pregnant women with complex or severe mental illness should be seen by a psychiatrist (if available, a specialist in perinatal psychiatry) as soon as possible after the pregnancy has been identified.

Women of childbearing potential

- Given the frequency of unplanned pregnancies, family planning should be discussed with all women with a mental illness who have childbearing potential. They should be informed about the effects of the prescribed psychotropic medication on the foetus and the effects of childbearing and not taking medication on their illness.
- Valproate and carbamazepine should not be offered for the treatment of psychiatric disorders. Women who plan a pregnancy and suffer from a severe or complex mental illness should be offered preconception counselling, if possible, by a perinatal psychiatrist. The considerations are the same as described for pregnancy in the next section.

Pregnancy

The decision about whether to continue psychotropic medication in pregnancy should be based on illness history, likely consequences, past treatment response, social and personal circumstances and the patient's informed attitude to the risk of stopping or continuing particular drugs.

Choice of medication

- The main principles are as follows:
  - Avoid drugs with higher risks of teratogenicity and other adverse child outcomes.
  - Use the individual patient's past history of effectiveness and tolerability of different medications to guide choice.

▨ *Mood stabilisers and lithium*
  - Other than in exceptional circumstances, valproate should be stopped regardless of the stage of pregnancy (see Chapter 5); it increases the rate of major congenital malformations threefold and raises the likelihood of intellectual impairment and autism spectrum disorder in the offspring.
  - Carbamazepine should be avoided based on limited evidence of efficacy and potential severity of neural tube defects.
  - High-dose folic acid at best only partially prevents foetal toxicity with valproate and carbamazepine.
  - Lithium is associated with a smaller risk of cardiovascular malformations than initially suggested, but if anomalies occur, they may be severe. It should only be used in the first trimester of pregnancy if no other medication is likely to be effective.
  - Lamotrigine does not appear to pose a major reproductive risk based on limited data.
▨ *Antidepressants*
  - Exposure in early pregnancy is associated with a small increase in the risk of major congenital malformations (mostly cardiovascular malformations), but causality is unclear. Paroxetine has been most consistently associated and should be avoided.
  - SSRIs (and probably serotonin and noradrenaline reuptake inhibitors) in late pregnancy increase the risk of persistent pulmonary hypertension of the newborn by about 2.5-fold, but from a very low base rate (about 1–2/1000).
  - Most antidepressants in late pregnancy treble the incidence of 'poor neonatal adaptation syndrome' (includes jitteriness, poor muscle tone, respiratory distress, hypoglycemia, low Apgar scores and seizures if severe); symptoms are usually mild and transient.
  - A causal association between autism spectrum disorder in the offspring and intrauterine exposure to SSRIs is unclear.
  - SSRIs are the preferred option if antidepressants need to be initiated in pregnancy; less is known about the reproductive safety of TCAs.
▨ *Antipsychotics*
  - Taken in pregnancy are associated with a small increase in the risk of cardiovascular (mainly septal) defects, but causality, clinical importance and differences between drugs remain uncertain.
  - Are associated with a two-fold increase in the incidence of gestational diabetes, but whether this is a direct medication effect is unclear.
  - Antipsychotics often have to be continued in women with schizophrenia because of the high risk of relapse; in women with bipolar disorder, they offer an alternative to mood stabilisers.

- *Benzodiazepines*
    - Taken during late pregnancy have been associated with neonatal morbidity, including withdrawal symptoms and the 'floppy baby syndrome'.
    - They should only be used for the short-term management of severe agitation and anxiety.
- *Coprescribed psychotropics* should be avoided where possible because of unknown risks to the foetus.

Dosing in pregnancy

- Although clinicians often reduce the dose of medication in pregnancy in order to reduce risk to the foetus, a subtherapeutic dose should be avoided because
    - It increases the risk of recurrence or deterioration
    - The benefits to the foetus are unknown
- Pregnancy-induced pharmacokinetic changes mean that
    - Lithium requires close monitoring, particularly in the last month of gestation, intrapartum and the early post-natal period, to avoid both underdosing and maternal and infant toxicity. Changes in renal clearance mean that Na^+ depletion should be avoided.
    - Lamotrigine concentrations should be monitored closely in pregnancy and the early post-natal weeks, due to increased, but highly variable, metabolism during pregnancy.

Breastfeeding

- Because of significant benefits to the infant, exclusive breastfeeding for the first 6 months after childbirth is generally strongly encouraged.
- Most drugs taken in therapeutic doses are compatible with breastfeeding.
- The exceptions are
    - Clozapine
    - Lithium
    - Carbamazepine
    - Benzodiazepines with long half-lives
- Mothers should be informed that babies usually receive much less drug during breastfeeding than during pregnancy, but uncertainty about potential adverse effects remains, and they should monitor their baby for side effects.
- There is a lack of information about the safety of breastfeeding when the mother takes several psychotropic drugs, and treatment decisions have to be made on an individual basis.

 **Bibliography**

Guidelines

General Medical Council. Good practice in prescribing and managing medicines and devices. 2013; http://www.gmc-uk.org/Prescribing_guidance.pdf_59055247.pdf.

National Institute for Health and Care Excellence. Medicines adherence: Involving patients in decisions about prescribed medicines and supporting adherence. *NICE Clinical Guideline 76.* 2009; http://www.nice.org.uk/guidance/cg76.

National Institute for Care and Health Excellence. Antenatal and postnatal mental health: Clinical management and service guidance. *NICE Clinical Guideline 192.* 2014; http://www.nice.org.uk/guidance/cg192.

National Institute for Health and Care Excellence. Diabetes in pregnancy: Management of diabetes and its complications from pre-conception to the postnatal period. *NICE Clinical Guideline 63.* 2008; http://www.nice.org.uk/guidance/cg63.

Royal College of Psychiatrists. Use of licensed medicines for unlicensed applications in psychiatric practice. College Report CR142. 2007; http://www.rcpsych.ac.uk/files/pdfversion/cr142.pdf.

Key references

American Academy of Paediatrics. Breastfeeding and the use of human milk. *Pediatrics* 2012; 129: e827–e841.

Baldwin DS, Kosky N. Off-label prescribing in psychiatric practice. *Adv Psychiat Treat.* 2007; 13: 414–422.

Cramer JA, Rosenheck R. Compliance with medication regimens for mental and physical disorders. *Psychiatr Serv.* 1998; 49: 196–201.

Demyttenaere K, Albert A, Mesters P et al. What happens with adverse events during 6 months of treatment with selective serotonin reuptake inhibitors? *J Clin Psychiatry.* 2005; 66: 859–863.

Grigoriadis S, VonderPorten EH, Mamisashvili L et al. Antidepressant exposure during pregnancy and congenital malformations: Is there an association? A systematic review and meta-analysis of the best evidence. *J Clin Psychiatry.* 2013; 74: e293–e308.

Haddad PM. Ten principles of good psychiatric prescribing. *Medicine.* 2012; 40: 674–675.

Haddad PM, Anderson IM. Recognising and managing antidepressant discontinuation symptoms. *Adv Psychiat Treat.* 2007; 13: 447–457.

Haddad PM, Brain C, Scott J. Nonadherence with antipsychotic medication in schizophrenia: Challenges and management strategies. *Patient Relat Outcome Meas.* 2014; 5: 43–62.

Haddad PM, Fleischhacker WW, Peuskens J et al. SMARTS (Systematic Monitoring of Adverse events Related to TreatmentS): The development of a pragmatic patient-completed checklist to assess antipsychotic drug side effects. *Ther Adv Psychopharmacol.* 2014; 4: 15–21.

Haddad PM, Sharma SG. Adverse effects of atypical antipsychotics: Differential risk and clinical implications. *CNS Drugs.* 2007; 21: 911–936.

Källén B, Borg N, Reis M. The use of central nervous system active drugs during pregnancy. *Pharmaceuticals.* 2013; 6: 1221–1286.

Taylor D, Paton C, Kapur S. *The Maudsley Prescribing Guidelines in Psychiatry*, 12th edn. Chichester, UK: John Wiley & Sons Ltd., 2015.

Wieck A. The use of anti-epileptic medication in women with affective disorders in early and late pregnancy and during breastfeeding. *Curr Wom Health Rev.* 2011; 7: 50–57.

Zimmerman M, Posternak M, Friedman M et al. Which factors influence psychiatrists' selection of antidepressants? *Am J Psychiatry.* 2004; 161: 1285–1289.

Further reading

Grigoriadis S, VonderPorten EH, Mamisashvili L et al. The effect of prenatal antidepressant exposure on neonatal adaptation: A systematic review and meta-analysis. *J Clin Psychiatry.* 2013; 74: e309–e320.

Grigoriadis S, VonderPorten EH, Mamisashvili L et al. Prenatal exposure to antidepressants and persistent pulmonary hypertension of the newborn: Systematic review and meta-analysis. *Br Med J.* 2014; 348: f6932.

Meador KJ, Loring DW. Prenatal valproate exposure is associated with autism spectrum disorder and childhood autism. *J Pediatr.* 2013; 163: 924.

McKnight RF, Adida M, Budge K et al. Lithium toxicity profile: A systematic review and meta-analysis. *Lancet.* 2012; 379(9817): 721–728.

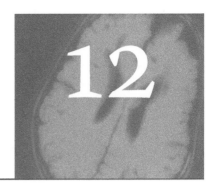

Clinical trial methodology

Stephen M Lawrie and
R Hamish McAllister-Williams

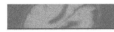 ## Introduction

- A general definition of 'clinical trial' is any kind of study designed to establish the effects of a particular therapeutic intervention.
- Table 10.1 gives some definitions of terminology used in trials.

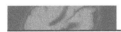 ## History

- Clinical trials of some sort are probably as old as civilisation.
- James Lind, an eighteenth-century Scottish physician, is generally credited with having completed the first controlled trial of vitamin C for scurvy.
- Early Nobel prizes awarded for interventions in the field of psychiatry, Wagner-Jauregg in 1927 for 'malaria therapy' and Moniz in 1949 for the prefrontal leucotomy, have proven to be ineffective and abused, respectively.
- The gold standard of medical experimentation, the randomised controlled trial (RCT), was first used to evaluate the effects of antituberculous drugs in a trial sponsored by the Medical Research Council and published in 1948.
- There is increasing interest in designing valid naturalistic or pragmatic trials to determine effectiveness in usual clinical practice.

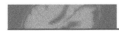 ## Drug development

- New drugs can be developed by
    - Isolating the active ingredients in natural compounds
    - Modifying the chemistry of other drugs
    - From theoretical extension of basic science knowledge

- Only about 1 in every 10,000 potential products reach the market, often taking 10 years or more and many millions of pounds. Given the limited patent life (20 years in the United Kingdom from the time of compound synthesis), drug companies often adopt aggressive marketing strategies to recoup their costs and deliver profits for shareholders.
- A new drug is first tested in animals, to establish potential for desired effects and absence of unexpected effects, before going through the four phases of drug development in humans (Table 12.1).
- *Phase I* trials determine basic pharmacological parameters in human volunteers, e.g. pharmacokinetics, adverse effects and tolerance
  - They are usually open or uncontrolled.
  - Adverse effects are often measured both subjectively and objectively (e.g. heart rate, blood pressure, neuropsychological performance, EEG).
  - Generally require 24 h clinical observations and often exclude the young, women and the old because the effects in humans are unknown; however, a drug safe in adult men, e.g. may not be safe in children, women and the aged.
  - Because studies are uncontrolled, some of the effects will be placebo effects.
- *Phase II* trials establish whether or not a given drug works in a variety of conditions
  - They are usually 'placebo-controlled', in that some patients get placebo.
  - In 'dose-ranging studies', each group of patients gets a particular dose of the drug to determine optimal dosage.
- *Phase III*, sometimes called 'comparative' trials, seeks to determine the effects of a new drug with reference to those commonly used in clinical practice
  - They are usually randomised with a proportion of patients receiving placebo (a variety of other types of trials may be randomised

Table 12.1 Phases of drug development

	Question addressed	Main methods
Preclinical	Pharmacology and toxicology	Biochemical and animal studies
Phase I	Basic human pharmacology	Open/uncontrolled
Phase II	Efficacy in disease(s)	Controlled trials/small randomised controlled trials
Phase III	Efficacy and comparative efficacy (for regulatory approval)	Randomised controlled trials
Phase IV	Problems in clinical practice/ comparison with other drugs	Observational studies/ randomised controlled trials

and/or controlled, but these are rarely used in drug development studies; see the following text).
  – They tend to be larger than Phase II studies.
  – Their major aim is to satisfy regulatory authorities and obtain a product licence.
- *Phase IV* clinical 'trials' refer to the various methods of surveillance (see the following text) to establish the frequency of any serious or unexpected adverse effects of a drug once it has been licensed and introduced into regular clinical practice.
  – They have similarities to audit (measuring performance against a standard) and naturalistic outcome studies (Table 12.3).

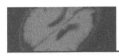

Designing or appraising a clinical trial (Table 12.2)

Clinical trials have traditionally been the preserve of experts, but increasingly there is a recognition, and requirement, for patient and public involvement (PPI) in the design and conduct of trials and in the implementation of their results.

Aim or hypothesis of the study

- Any study has a better chance of answering a single specific question rather than a number of less focused objectives. The question should be
  – Clinically relevant (i.e. the answer will help make therapeutic decisions)
  – Ethically acceptable (see Ethical considerations section)
  – Not answered already (e.g. in a large study or good quality systematic review and meta-analysis)

Table 12.2 Questions relating to the design or appraisal of a clinical trial

1. What is the aim or hypothesis of the study?
2. Which patients are being studied?
3. What intervention is being studied?
4. What type of clinical trial is appropriate?
5. Was randomisation appropriately carried out?
6. Which outcomes should be measured and how?
7. Were appropriate statistical tests used?

Nature of the patients being studied

- This is stipulated in inclusion and exclusion criteria.
- There is theoretical tension between recruiting a 'pure' highly selected group and an unselected heterogeneous group. The former reduces variance in the data and hence can produce more reliable results, but the findings may not be representative of the entire patient population. The latter may be more valid but it may be difficult to identify a given effect.
- In practice, broader inclusion criteria, and minimal exclusions, aid recruitment.
- Many psychiatric studies exclude patients with comorbid substance abuse or other disorders, which comprise about half of all the patients seen clinically. This
  - Leaves uncertainty about efficacy in the comorbid group
  - Probably overestimates the benefits of any treatment in practice (due to noncompliance and/or ineffectiveness being higher in comorbid patients)
- The usual practice of excluding patients <16–18 and >60–65 years of age means that they often have to be treated without information from clinical trials and 'off licence'.
- Involuntarily detained patients cannot usually be enrolled in clinical trials for ethical reasons. This means that the most severely ill patients may be treated in the absence of specific evidence for them (although treatment efficacy in specific disorders does not of course depend on legal status).
- The trial setting determines the type of patients to whom the results will apply (inpatients, outpatients and/or those in primary care).

Intervention being studied

- Consider the type, formulation, dose, dosing schedule and route of administration of the medication.
- *Fixed versus flexible dosing*
  - Results from fixed-dose trials are generally easier to interpret but are different from how a drug is used in clinical practice, and many patients will receive non-optimal doses.
  - Results from flexible dosing (tailoring the dose to a particular patient) are more clinically representative but can be difficult if the responsible clinician is blind to the treatment given.
- What, if any, other drugs are permissible for participating patients, e.g. antipsychotic trials usually permit anticholinergic drugs for extra pyramidal side effects and 'rescue' medication for behavioural disturbance.
- *Comparator/s*
  - Having a placebo comparison is desirable to establish efficacy and also if against an active comparator to show whether the study is able to show a treatment effect.

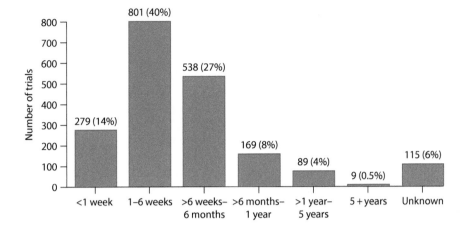

Figure 12.1 Duration of the first 2000 clinical trials in schizophrenia. (Reproduced by permission from Thornley B and Adams C. *BMJ* 1998; 317: 1181.)

- Consider whether the choice, and dose, of any comparator is appropriate for the aims of the study.
■ *Duration*
  - Most efficacy trials have been short (6 weeks or less) simply because they are easier to do (Figure 12.1). Longer trials have become more common (e.g. for depression, anxiety disorders).
  - Long trials are expensive and liable to have large numbers of people dropping out. The more dropouts, the less reliable are the results of the trial (but it is hard to avoid dropouts in many psychiatric studies).
■ Ideally, clinical practice should be informed by long-term clinical trials, particularly if advising patients to stay on a drug for 1 year or more. However, this needs to be balanced against the likelihood of higher dropout rates, and difficulty maintaining allocated treatment (e.g. against placebo), which can compromise the validity of the study.

Types of clinical trials (Table 12.3)

■ *Uncontrolled trials*
  - Can indicate whether a treatment works at all and the profile of adverse effects.
  - However, non-specific/placebo effects cannot be excluded without a control group.
■ *Controlled trials*
  - Allow evaluation against placebo or a pre-existing treatment.
  - May reduce or control for placebo effects.

Table 12.3 Some commonly used terms to describe types of trials

Term	Meaning
Controlled	A group receiving the investigative treatment is compared with another group receiving different treatment (e.g. placebo, no treatment or waiting list, another treatment of known efficacy). Usually applied to *prospective* (i.e. both groups are studied in parallel) rather than *retrospective* (i.e. using a historical control group treated at a previous time) trials.
Placebo-controlled	One of the 'arms' of the trial is against a placebo condition. Usually required for a drug to be licensed.
Randomised	Allocation to the different treatment 'arms' in the study is done randomly to minimise bias due to selection of patients for particular treatments.
Open	Both clinician and patient know that a treatment is being given for a given indication. Open studies are usually uncontrolled. (NB: In clinical practice this is often equivalent to giving a therapeutic trial for an unlicensed indication.)
Single-blind	Usually taken to indicate that the assessing clinicians, but not the patients, are informed about which treatment is being given.[a]
Double-blind	Neither the patient nor the assessing clinician is informed of which treatment is being given.[a]
Triple-blind	Sometimes used when there are separate treating clinicians and assessors, both of whom, as well as the patient, are blind to treatment allocation.[a]
Naturalistic/pragmatic	Trials carried out in usual clinical practice with trade-off between rigorous trial methodology and 'real-world' applicability.
Non-inferiority	Trials statistically powered to be able to detect a pre-specified difference between two active drugs that is judged to be clinically significant.

[a] It is usually not checked/made clear whether blinding is successful in practice.

- – In the absence of randomisation, they are still subject to selection bias (conscious or unconscious). Patients who get a new treatment tend to be less ill and/or have better prognosis. Without randomisation, the benefits of new drugs are typically overestimated by 30%–40%.
- ▪ *RCTs* were devised to measure drug efficacy and probably offer the greatest precision. They measure how well a drug works in ideal conditions. However, they are not without problems and alternative approaches may be sufficient or optimum, depending on the specific clinical question.

- Randomisation increases the scientific quality or 'internal validity' of a trial (see the Randomisation section).
- Typically assessment of outcome is 'blinded' (see the Outcomes and measurement section and Table 12.3).
- There are, however, problems with 'external validity', i.e. patients able to give informed consent and willing to be randomised tend to differ from many potential participants. This limits their representativeness and reduces generalisability of the results.
- Establishing the efficacy of a drug requires RCTs designed to show a greater effect than placebo (with sufficient statistical power).
- RCTs against comparator drugs are frequently underpowered to be able to show a difference, so claims of equal efficacy need to be treated with caution. This has led to the development of *non-inferiority* studies. These are designed to have sufficient statistical power to detect a predefined difference between drugs, which is believed to be of clinical importance (see 'Power calculation' in the following text).
- *Pragmatic (or naturalistic) trials* measure clinical effectiveness (how well a drug works in usual clinical practice). They are increasingly being applied in psychiatry:
  - They have more external, but less internal, validity than RCTs.
  - Patient groups are representative, the interventions are routinely feasible, outcome measures are clinically relevant and usually other treatments are allowed as clinically indicated.
  - The emphasis is on assessment by initial randomisation group.
- *Patient preference trials*
  - Are a specific type of pragmatic trial.
  - Patients not willing to be randomised are given their preferred treatment. They are followed up as in the trial and their results are compared with randomised patients.
- *Crossover trials*
  - All participants receive two (or more) interventions one after the other, with the two groups receiving a different treatment first.
  - Useful in relatively rare diseases where small numbers do not permit an RCT.
  - However, it is difficult to ensure that the trial is long enough to see therapeutic effects but short enough to avoid natural fluctuations confounding the trial.
  - There is the problem of carry-over effects from the first treatment period to the second and the potential for drug interactions.
  - 'Washout periods' of no treatment introduce new difficulties with sudden cessation of potentially effective treatments.
- *N-of-1 trials*
  - Are crossover trials in which a patient is given two treatments. May be useful if it is not known which treatment they may benefit from.
  - Require patient consent and cooperation from the hospital pharmacy.

▦ *Audit and naturalistic outcome studies*
   – Not usually thought of as clinical trials but are similar to Phase IV 'trials'.
   – Provide valuable effectiveness information, but are uncontrolled and therefore of reduced internal validity even if patients are used as their own 'historical control' (called *mirror-image studies* when periods before and after an intervention are compared).

Randomisation

▦ There are two main purposes of randomisation:
   – To evenly distribute known and unknown confounders (e.g. age, sex, prognostic factors) affecting outcome.
   – To avoid selection bias (which depends on concealing allocation).
▦ Successful randomisation is inversely related to the chance of a trial finding a treatment effect (in one review, 58% of randomised studies, where allocation could have been compromised, found a benefit of the new treatment, versus 9% of randomised trials with adequate allocation concealment).
▦ *Allocation concealment in randomisation*
   – Is different to blinding (Table 12.3).
   – Requires unpredictable randomisation schedule (i.e. not dates of birth, day of admission to hospital); otherwise, investigators may consciously or unconsciously subvert randomisation.
▦ *Randomisation consists of*
   – Assignment at random (coin tossing is an acceptable way of generating the schedule).
   – Treatment assignment only revealed after consent to participate obtained (preferably by independent person).
   – Methods include sealed opaque envelopes, telephoning centralised allocation unit.
▦ Randomisation can include methods to ensure that trial groups are balanced in terms of number and/or patient characteristics:
   – '*Blocked*' in groups (of 4, 6, etc. or variable numbers) to ensure broadly equal numbers in groups.
   – '*Stratified*' to ensure possible prognostic factors (e.g. age, sex, duration of illness) are balanced; this requires a randomisation schedule for each stratum.
   – '*Minimisation*' in which subsequent patients are allocated by minimising differences in important variables; requires a computerised system.
▦ Cluster trials are those in which subjects are randomised in groups or clusters, most common for wider aspects of health services than one

particular treatment (e.g. effects of education on general practitioners done by group practice). The main disadvantage is that the unit of randomisation should be the unit of analysis requiring large numbers of individuals for adequate power.

Outcomes and measurement

▨ Outcomes need to be valid and reliable and relevant to the aims of the study.

▨ There is increasing emphasis on outcomes being relevant to patient experience.

▨ However, outcome measures in trials of drug treatment have changed relatively little over the years, partly driven by the need in commercial trials to meet the requirements of regulatory authorities for product licensing.

▨ Clinical outcomes can be measured either categorically (e.g. recovered/ not recovered) or continuously (e.g. symptom severity scales).

▨ *Categorical outcomes*
  – Are easiest to understand and are potentially the most clinically meaningful
  – May be determined from arbitrary cut-off points on rating scales or other measures (e.g. response measured as a percentage reduction in symptom severity)
  – Require non-parametric statistics

▨ *Outcomes*
  – Should be pre-specified as primary (ideally one) and secondary (can be many).
  – Typically are symptom severity scores, but might include adverse effects, dropouts and quality-of-life measures.
  – Multiple outcome measures increase finding significant differences by chance, unless statistical adjustments are made.

▨ *Rating scales*
  – If observer-rated scales are used, these should be reliable (when rated by two or more observers) and should be sensitive to change.
  – Psychiatry has had a surfeit of rating scales making comparison between trials problematic.
  – Researchers who use self-devised scales are more likely to report statistically significant effects than if they use standard measures.
  – Self-rated questionnaires are increasingly being used as they avoid observer bias. However, this does not mean that any participant-related measurement errors are eliminated.
  – There is interest in using patient-reported outcome measures (PROMs) better tailored to patient experience and priorities.

- ▨ *Blinding*
  - – Aims to reduce bias and placebo effects (Table 12.3).
  - – Is rarely entirely successful (response or side effects may reveal which treatment has been given), especially if the primary outcome measure is 'soft' (subjective) as opposed to 'hard' (e.g. death or hospital admission).
  - – Independent outcome assessors may mitigate these problems to some degree.
  - – May not be possible in participants of some treatments (e.g. psychological treatments).
  - – Success of blinding can be estimated by asking participants/ assessors which treatment they think was received. However, interpretation may be complicated by participants equating success with active treatment when there is a large benefit, rather than because the blind was broken.

Statistical issues

- ▨ *Effect size, significance and importance*
  - – Care should be taken to distinguish between *statistical significance* and *clinical importance* (Note: 'Clinical significance' is often used but best avoided as it tends to elide the two meanings).
  - – Clinical importance relates to the magnitude of the *effect size* in practice (e.g. is the advantage of the drug over placebo big enough to be clinically relevant?).
  - – The effect size needed to reach clinical importance may be arbitrarily determined (e.g. for depression the NICE (2004) guideline defined this to be three points on the Hamilton Depression Rating scale for first-line antidepressant treatment versus placebo; it was abandoned as too rigid in the NICE 2009 guideline update, but has 'stuck' and is frequently reiterated).
  - – The smaller the effect size, the larger the sample needed to have a chance of detecting a statistically significant effect (see 'Power calculation' in the following text). Beware of large samples with statistically significant but clinically irrelevant findings. (NB: On its own, the size of the P-value does not indicate the effect size or clinical importance.)
  - – It has been argued that because of large (and increasing) placebo response rates in RCTs, and the highly selected patients enrolled, the only meaningful way of assessing the clinical effect size of an intervention is through large pragmatic studies. RCTs may only indicate statistical difference rather than clinical importance.
- ▨ *Power calculation*
  - – Is necessary to determine the number of participants needed to detect a given finding at a specified level of statistical

significance. This requires a defined primary outcome measure with estimation of numbers achieving a categorical outcome or a likely mean difference on a continuous measure given its likely variance.

- It is standard to aim for 90% power (80% is often acceptable) to detect a given effect size with P < 0.05 difference, but different values can be specified. Various methods are available to calculate this, e.g. tables, computerised statistical packages, web-based calculators.

Size of trial

- Most early RCTs in depression or schizophrenia had less than 60 participants (Figure 12.2). This is often inadequate to identify significant differences between an active treatment and placebo but depends on the effect size.
- Trials comparing two active agents require much larger groups as the difference is generally much smaller.
- Larger trials measure outcomes more accurately because the patients are likely to be more representative, measurement error is reduced and they tend to be better planned and organised.
- Very large (mega) trials, including thousands of patients, are the best way of answering important therapeutic questions, but there is a risk that small, clinically insignificant differences will be found.

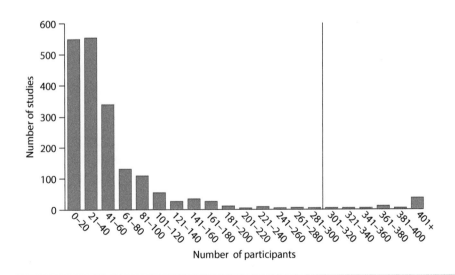

Figure 12.2 The size of the first 2000 controlled trials in schizophrenia. The line indicates the number of patients required to find a 20% difference between treatments with standard power. (Reproduced by permission from Thornley B and Adams C. *BMJ* 1998; 317: 1181.)

Missing data
  – All clinical trials will have missing data. Two important features are the amount of data missing (if it is large it limits applicability of the trial) and how it is missing.
  – *Missing completely at random (MCAR)* means that the likelihood of data being missing is unrelated to any study variables and results in no bias.
  – *Missing at random (MAR)* means that the missing data are dependent on observed study variables (e.g. severity, age, sex) but not on the values of the missing data. This is common and can be accounted for by covarying for the observed values and if predicable may be addressed in study design (e.g. stratification).
  – *Missing not at random (MNAR)* means that whether or not data are missing depends on their values, and this will bias the results.
■ *Types of analysis*
  – The appropriate statistical tests needed depend on the properties of the data.
  – Continuous measures provide more statistical power than categorical ones, but the latter can have advantages when dealing with dropouts from the trial (see the following text).
  – *Completer analysis* includes only those who are still in the trial at the end. Overestimates treatment effects and is generally to be avoided.
  – *Intention-to-treat (ITT)* analyses all randomised participants, i.e. including trial dropouts. With categorical measures, dropouts can be conservatively assumed to have had a poor outcome. This may under- or overestimate efficacy and is difficult to interpret if there is a high rate of dropouts, or if the rate differs between treatments.
  – *Last observation carried forward (LOCF)* analysis has been the standard approach with a continuous measure, using the last available measure as the final measure, but is being superseded by alternative ways of dealing with missing data. LOCF may be ITT if includes baseline data; alternatively it may only include subjects who have completed a certain period of treatment (e.g. 2 weeks). May over- or underestimate efficacy.
  – *Multiple imputation* or *likelihood-based* analyses have been used to give a better estimate of outcome than the traditional LOCF approach. The likelihood-based *mixed effects model repeated measures (MMRM)* models the time course for missing data rather than carrying forward the last value unchanged. It may reduce both under- and overestimates of treatment effect with LOCF analysis.
  – It is desirable that ITT analyses make plausible assumptions about missing data (see earlier text) and include sensitivity analyses of departures from these assumptions.

▪ *Problematic analyses*
  - The success of randomisation should not be tested by comparing descriptive variables; some will differ by chance.
  - Defining subgroups of patients by who responded particularly well or badly to treatment and taking this to indicate that certain groups should get particular treatments. The exception is if there was a pre-specified *a priori* hypothesis. Post hoc subgroup analysis is acceptable if clearly presented as exploratory, i.e. for future hypothesis testing.
  - *Multiple hypothesis testing.* One statistical comparison in 20 is likely to be significant at $P < 0.05$ by chance alone. It is acceptable if there are pre-specified hypotheses, but correction for multiple testing should be made. Exploratory testing ('data dredging') is acceptable if clearly stated as such.
▪ *Meta-analysis*
  - Individual RCTs are prone to bias, random variation and type II errors. *Meta-analysis* pools results from individual studies to increase power.
  - It must be part of a systematic review to attempt to get all relevant studies to avoid selection bias; nevertheless, publication bias remains possible as negative RCTs may be unpublished, especially if small.
  - New methods including *mega-analysis* (using individual patient data from different studies), and *network*, or *mixed-methods, meta-analysis* (combining both comparative and non-comparative studies) are becoming increasingly popular.
  - It must be remembered that the quality of the studies, methods of study selection, data extraction and subsequent combination can vary tremendously and will greatly influence the conclusions drawn and the validity of the results. There are examples where a rigorous, sufficiently large, RCT has overturned the results from a meta-analysis.
  - Evidence-based medicine projects such as the Cochrane Collaboration aim to improve the registration of clinical trials and the synthesis of results (http://www.cochrane.org).

Non-specific effects

▪ Studies are inescapably confounded by non-specific effects which lead to improvement in the absence of any specific pharmacological action of the drug being studied.
▪ Response rates on placebo can be very high (typically 30%–40% in 8-week antidepressant or antipsychotic studies).
▪ Placebo response rates in depression positively correlate with the year of study publication, that is, rates are increasing. This is likely to apply

262 Fundamentals of Clinical Psychopharmacology

to other disorders and may relate to increasing use of more mildly ill patients (see the following text).

▨ These may lead to
  – Incorrect assumption of efficacy in uncontrolled trials.
  – Incorrect assumption of inefficacy in underpowered studies due to type II statistical errors ('false negatives').
  – Questioning of clinical importance, even if statistical significance is attained, as a high response rate to placebo tends to lead to smaller effect sizes (against placebo).

▨ There are three main components to the non-specific response: Measurement effects, placebo effects and spontaneous recovery.

▨ *Measurement effects*
  – When a population is chosen for a characteristic above a cut-off (e.g. psychiatric rating scale score > x), then a second measurement will tend to be less simply because of imperfect reliability in measurement (called *regression to the mean*).
  – *Observer expectations*: Rating values may be elevated to include patients in a trial; subsequent ratings may be more accurate or lowered by expecting improvement. These can lead to bias if treatment allocation is known and expectations vary between treatment arms.
  – *Participant demand characteristics*: Rating values may be influenced by wish to meet assessor expectations. This may potentially lead to bias if treatment allocation is known. Knowledge of treatment is unavoidable with psychological treatments.

▨ *Placebo effects (genuine, but non-specific, treatment effects)*
  – In RCTs, patients assigned to the placebo arm have regular visits and support. This constitutes a treatment in its own right.
  – Patient (and doctor or researcher) expectations may engage a non-pharmacological healing process. This factor may be more potent in less ill patients and in those with greater motivation (e.g. recruited from advertisements).
  – Placebo effects are intrinsic to psychological treatments, and some argue that teasing them out from specific effects is not appropriate. However, this makes comparisons (especially indirect ones) of the size of intervention effect of drug and psychological RCTs problematic.

▨ *Spontaneous recovery*
  – This reflects the natural history of the disorder. It is likely to be greater in more mildly ill patients with shorter length of illness.

Ethical considerations

▨ Ethical issues apply to all stages of any trial. The Declaration of Helsinki (7th revision) applies (see Guidelines).

▧ *Planning a trial*
 – The trial should address an unresolved question.
 – It should use methods likely to provide a useful answer, e.g. be sufficiently powered.
 – A specific issue has been the ethics of placebo control in conditions such as schizophrenia and depression where standard treatments are effective.
 – Attention needs to be paid to what treatment is offered at the termination of the trial, particularly if patients have been treated with placebo.
 – Ethical approval is required with patient information and consent forming an important aspect of the application.
 – Drugs unlicensed for a particular indication need specific trial approval from the regulatory authorities (MHRA in the United Kingdom) with regulations implementing the EU Directive on Good Clinical Practice in Clinical Trials (2001) (see Guidelines).

▧ *Consent*
 – Fully informed, usually written, consent is required; participants should fully appreciate the nature of the trial and the potential risks and benefits.
 – May be a particular problem in psychiatry, e.g. in dementia and psychosis. Cognitive impairment may be amenable to appropriately structured informed consent procedures.
 – Third-party consent may be appropriate good practice if a participant cannot consent or lacks capacity, but lacks legal force and is likely to reduce enrolment.

▧ *Conduct of the trial*
 – Good clinical practice (GCP) guidelines apply, e.g. MHRA guidance and EU directives.
 – Payment or inducement is not generally allowed, but compensation can be given, e.g. for travel and subsistence. Healthy volunteers can also receive compensation for inconvenience or discomfort.
 – Insurance or indemnity agreement may be necessary for adverse effects.
 – Research data are confidential and should be stored anonymously and safely.

▧ Fraudulent analysis or presentation of results of a trial is unethical and may be misleading or dangerous.

▧ Ethical structures and procedures are continuing to evolve and it is important to keep up to date. In the United Kingdom, Ethics Committees are legally accountable to the Health Research Authority (http://www.hra.nhs.uk/), and there is a unified web-based application system. There remains debate about the balance to be struck between protecting research subjects and increased restrictions and bureaucracy discouraging research.

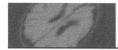

Post-marketing surveillance/ Phase IV clinical trials

Some important adverse effects detected by post-marketing surveillance are shown in Table 12.4.

Voluntary reporting

- Depends upon the observational skills and conscientiousness of individual clinicians.
- Countries have national reporting systems. In the United Kingdom, the MHRA encourage notification of possible adverse reactions, especially for new products (indicated by 'black triangles'), by professionals and patients using the 'Yellow Card Scheme' (https://yellowcard.mhra.gov.uk/).
- National centres can send such information to the WHO Collaborating Centre for International Drug Monitoring.

Table 12.4 Some important adverse effects detected by post-marketing surveillance

Year	Drug	Adverse effect
1961	Thalidomide	Phocomelia[a]
1963	MAOIs	Cheese (hypertensive) reactions
1976	Clozapine	Agranulocytosis[b]
1979–1990	Mianserin	Blood dyscrasia[b]
1983	Zimelidine	Hypersensitivity reactions and Guillain–Barré syndrome[a]
1986	Nomifensine	Haemolytic anaemia[a]
1990	Pimozide	Ventricular arrhythmias[b]
1993	Remoxipride	Aplastic anaemia[a]
1998	Sertindole	Possibility of sudden (cardiac) death[a]
1999	Vigabatrin	Visual field defects[b]
2001	Droperidol	QT prolongation on ECG[a]
2001 (2005)	Thioridazine	QT prolongation on ECG[b] (United Kingdom[a])
2003	Nefazodone	Hepatotoxicity[a] (United States[b])
2008	Rimonabant	Depression and suicide[a]

[a] Leading to product withdrawal (or highly restricted use).
[b] Leading to requirements for appropriate monitoring (and usually restricted use as well).

- *The method*
  - Is cheap and has identified adverse effects resulting in withdrawal of particular products, e.g. remoxipride
  - Probably underestimates serious adverse effects and is inadequate as an epidemiological tool

Intensive surveillance

- More intensive surveillance is expensive and usually restricted to hospital inpatients.
- Examples include the Boston Collaborative Drug Surveillance Programme (http://www.bu.edu/bcdsp) and the Tayside Medicines Monitoring Unit (MEMO) in the United Kingdom (http://www.dundee.ac.uk/memo/).

Retrospective studies

- These are more expensive, but much more informative, than simple voluntary systems.
- Drawbacks are those of selection bias and unavailability of information.
- *Examples include*
  - Simple case-control studies
  - Pre-existing data storage systems, such as the Office of Population Censuses and Surveys (OPCS) data
  - The UK-based Clinical Practice Research Database (it reported an increased risk of venous thromboembolism on antipsychotic drugs)
- Databases can be linked by computer, e.g. people exposed to a particular product or people admitted to hospital with a particular problem. Linking a national registry of clozapine recipients to national death records found that clozapine increased the risk of fatal pulmonary embolism and respiratory disorders but reduced the risk of suicide.

Prospective studies

- These are the most reliable but also the most expensive.
- *Examples are*
  - A new product may be released with recorded/registered prescriptions to facilitate monitoring.
  - An established product can be monitored, e.g. prompted blood tests with clozapine.
  - Prescription event monitoring (PEM), now evolved into modified-PEM, or M-PEM, in England, aims to prospectively assess events occurring in 1000 patients prescribed a drug. Prescribing data are matched with questionnaires sent to general practitioners in which

they record demographics, medication, prescribing information, clinical events and pregnancy. This is being extended to a specialist cohort event monitoring (SCEM) scheme, initially for asenapine.

 ## Conclusions

- Patients need protection from unscrupulous or overenthusiastic trialists, but trials are needed to establish the efficacy and effectiveness of new treatments.
- The 'explanatory' RCT has given clinical therapeutics a sound scientific base but measures efficacy rather than effectiveness.
- Pragmatic clinical trials and multicentre studies in psychiatry are still at an early stage but have much to commend them in determining effectiveness in clinical practice.
- Single trials can be cited to prove virtually anything, and results need independent replication.
- Systematic reviews and meta-analyses can reliably synthesise available evidence but are no better than the studies they contain.
- Psychiatrists have been overreliant on the pharmaceutical industry to evaluate new products and need to conduct more independent large/mega trials. However, funding such studies is problematic.

Bibliography

Guidelines

European Union Directive 2001/20/EC on Good Clinical Practice in Clinical Trials (see http://www.mhra.gov.uk for details and current consultation on their implementation).

Medicines and Healthcare Products Regulatory Agency. Good clinical practice for clinical trials. 2014; https://www.gov.uk/good-clinical-practice-for-clinical-trials.

World Medical Association Declaration of Helsinki. Ethical Principles for Medical Research Involving Human Subjects (7th revision). 2013; http://www.wma.net/en/30publications/10policies/b3/index.html.

Key references

Carpenter WT Jr, Gold JM, Lahti AC et al. Decisional capacity for informed consent in schizophrenia research. *Arch Gen Psychiatry.* 2000; 57: 533–538.

Chalmers TC, Celano P, Sacks HS, Smith H Jr. Bias in treatment assignment in controlled clinical trials. *N Engl J Med.* 1983; 309: 1358–1361.

Even C, Siobud-Dorocant E, Dardennes RM. Critical approach to antidepressant trials. Blindness protection is necessary, feasible and measurable. *Br J Psychiatry.* 2000; 177: 47–51.

Louis TA, Lavori PW, Bailar JCD, Polansky M. Crossover and self-controlled designs in clinical research. *N Engl J Med.* 1984; 310: 24–31.

Marshall M, Lockwood A, Bradley C et al. Unpublished rating scales: A major source of bias in randomised controlled trials of treatments for schizophrenia. *Br J Psychiatry.* 2000; 176: 249–252.

Schulz KF, Chalmers I, Hayes RJ, Altman DG. Empirical evidence of bias. Dimensions of methodological quality associated with estimates of treatment effects in controlled trials. *JAMA.* 1995; 273: 408–412.

Schulz KF, Altman DG, Moher D, for the CONSORT Group. CONSORT 2010 statement: Updated guidelines for reporting parallel group randomised trials. *BMJ.* 2010; 340: 698–702.

Thornley B, Adams C. Content and quality of 2000 controlled trials in schizophrenia over 50 years. *BMJ.* 1998; 317: 1181–1184.

Walker AM, Lanza LL, Arellano F, Rothman KJ. Mortality in current and former users of clozapine. *Epidemiology.* 1997; 8: 671–677.

White IR, Horton NJ, Carpenter J, Pocock SJ. Strategy for intention to treat analysis in randomised trials with missing outcome data. *BMJ.* 2011; 342: 910–912.

Wood L, Egger M, Gluud LL et al. Empirical evidence of bias in treatment effect estimates in controlled trials with different interventions and outcomes: Meta-epidemiological study. *BMJ.* 2008; 336: 601–605.

Zornberg GL, Jick H. Antipsychotic drug use and risk of first-time idiopathic venous thromboembolism: A case-control study. *Lancet.* 2000; 356: 1219–1223.

Further reading

Edwards IR, Aronson JK. Adverse drug reactions: Definitions, diagnosis, and management. *Lancet.* 2000; 356: 1255–1259.

Everitt B, Wessely S. *Clinical Trials in Psychiatry.* Oxford, UK: Oxford University Press, 2004.

Friedman LM, Furberg, CD, DeMets DL. *Fundamentals of Clinical Trials.* New York: Springer, 2010.

Guyatt G, Sackett D, Taylor DW et al. Determining optimal therapy—Randomized trials in individual patients. *N Engl J Med.* 1986; 314: 889–892.

Lawrie SM, McIntosh AM, Rao S. *Critical Appraisal for Psychiatry.* Edinburgh, UK: Churchill Livingstone, 2000.

McIntosh AM, Sharpe M, Lawrie SM. Research methods statistics and evidence-based practice. In *Companion to Psychiatric Studies*, Johnstone EC, Cunningham Owens D, Lawrie SM, McIntosh AM and Sharpe M (eds.) 8th edn. Edinburgh, UK: Churchill Livingstone, 2010; pp 157–198.

Index

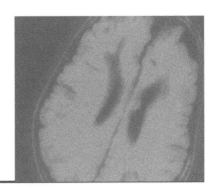